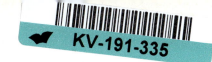

WHO Regional Publications, European Series, No. 54

Economic change, social welfare and health in Europe

Edited by
Lowell S. Levin
Laurie McMahon
Erio Ziglio

World Health Organization
Regional Office for Europe
Copenhagen

ISBN 92 890 1318 4
ISSN 0378-2255

The Regional Office for Europe of the World Health Organization welcomes requests for permission to reproduce or translate its publications, in part or in full. Applications and enquiries should be addressed to the Office of Publications, WHO Regional Office for Europe, Scherfigsvej 8, DK-2100 Copenhagen Ø, Denmark, which will be glad to provide the latest information on any changes made to the text, plans for new editions, and reprints and translations already available.

PRINTED IN FINLAND

CONTENTS

Contributors

Johan Fritzell has a Ph.D. in sociology, and is Associate Professor of Sociology at the Swedish Institute for Social Research. His main research interests have been income distribution and social policy. Recent publications include an international comparison of trends in income inequality, as well as analyses of welfare trends in Sweden during the 1980s. He is also co-director of the Swedish Level of Living project.

Sakari Hänninen has a Ph.D. in political science and is a researcher in the Social Research Unit of the National Research and Development Centre for Welfare and Health, in Helsinki. He has recently studied the consequences of the continuing economic depression for social policies in Finland.

Matti Heikkila has a Ph.D. in sociology and is Head of the Social Research Unit in the National Research and Development Centre for Welfare and Health, in Helsinki. His main research interest has been the issues of poverty and deprivation in the welfare state context. Recently, he has led a research project that explores the consequences of economic stagnation for welfare policies in Finland.

Osmo Kontula has a Ph.D. in sociology and is Research Director at the Department of Public Health, University of Helsinki. His research interests have been sexual behaviour among adults and adolescents, the use of illicit drugs and related policies, and the effect on health of economic depression. He has published over 20 books.

Kaj Koskela, MD, M.Sc., M.Pol.Sc., Ph.D., is a medical doctor and a sociologist. He holds the position of Permanent Counsellor at the Ministry of Social Affairs and Health in Finland. His research has centred around public health, disease prevention and health education. Recent publications include an analysis of the effects of the economic recession on health in Finland.

Eero Lahelma has a Ph.D. in sociology and is Associate Professor of Medical Sociology at the Department of Public Health, University of Helsinki. He has done research on employment, unemployment and health, and social inequalities in health. Recent work has included comparative analyses of health inequalities among men and women in Finland, other Scandinavian countries and Great Britain. He is Director of the Research Group on the Social Patterning of Health.

Olle Lundberg has a Ph.D in sociology, and is Associate Professor of Sociology at the Swedish Institute for Social Research. His research has been centred around the social causes of disease, with a special focus on health inequalities between social classes, as well as between men and women. Recent work has included analyses of welfare trends in Sweden during the 1980s, childhood conditions and adult health, and the importance of a sense of coherence for health.

Peter Makara has a Ph.D. in sociology and is Scientific Director of the National Institute for Health Promotion, Budapest, Hungary. He is also Director of the WHO Collaborating Centre for the Action Plan on Tobacco, national coordinator for the European Network of Health Promoting Schools and for two World Bank projects in the public health field, Deputy Chairman of the Hungarian Public Health Society and Visiting Professor at the University of Debrecen. His research has been centred around the social causes of disease, health promotion and health policy assessment.

Laurie McMahon is Director of Organisational Consultancy at the Office for Public Management, and has extensive experience in management and organizational learning. He has managed action research programmes associated with large-scale organizational change, has been a postgraduate teacher and consultant, both in the United Kingdom and overseas; and has run programmes for top management in the National Health Service. Laurie has degrees in behavioural sciences from the University of Aston and policy analysis from the University of Bristol. His main interests are in strategy development and implementation, organizational design, and the use of management games and simulations as aids to organizational learning. He is a trustee of the Public Management Foundation.

Leo Niskanen is docent in internal medicine and is Senior Lecturer at the University of Kuopio. His research interests have been related to epidemiology and, more recently, the metabolic and cardiovascular aspects of glucose tolerance and nutrition. Recent work has also included analyses on the effects of unemployment on mental wellbeing.

Heimo Viinamäki has an M.Sc.D. in psychiatry and is Assistant Senior Physician in the Department of Psychiatry at Kuopio University Hospital. His research has centred around general hospital psychiatry and the psychodynamic theory of health education. Recent work has included an analysis of outcome in psychiatric treatment and the mental health status of the unemployed.

Margaret Whitehead is a biologist, who had a background in medical and health education research before becoming an independent consultant. Her special interests include inequalities in health, in relation to which she has published *The health divide* (an update of the Black report). Recent work has included discussion documents on equity in health for WHO, and an analysis of the equity implications of the National Health Service reforms in the United Kingdom. She is currently a Visiting Fellow of the King's Fund Institute in London.

Wolfgang Zapf is Professor of Sociology at the Free University in Berlin and President of the Social Science Centre, Berlin (WZB). His research concentrates on modernization and welfare development in modern societies, recently with an emphasis on transformation in eastern and western Germany. He is co-director of the German welfare surveys.

Foreword

Powerful economic changes are having a profound effect, both positive and negative, on people's opportunities for health and the general quality of their lives in the WHO European Region. Understanding the origins, complexity, and far-reaching implications of these changes is a prerequisite for building public policies that will protect and develop the wellbeing of all Europeans, in accordance with target 13 of the regional strategy for health for all, on healthy public policy. Economists, sociologists, behavioural scientists and public health experts must pool their opinions and analyses to reveal fresh insights and possibilities for intervention. We must move from purely theoretical discourse towards a strategy for action, based on a policy for investing in health.

To further these aims, the WHO Regional Office for Europe joined the Finnish National Research and Development Centre for Welfare and Health to sponsor an international symposium on the social determinants of health: The Effects of Economic Changes on Social Welfare and Health. The 30 participants, from northern and central Europe, the United States and Zambia, contributed their ideas and views in a way that clarified the options for action. While they did not expect to reach consensus on all the key points discussed, they agreed strongly on the values and principles involved, on the needs for additional information and research, and on a general agenda for action.

Both at national and international levels, the discussions clearly revealed how much work lies ahead, particularly in closing the information gaps, in monitoring key economic and social changes with short- and long-term impact on health, and in evaluating data on intervention alternatives. Research and development organizations such as the Finnish National Research and Development Centre for Welfare and Health can play a central role as a stimulus, focal point, and information disseminator at the national level. The WHO Regional Office for Europe stands ready to extend the benefits of such centres throughout the Region by further strengthening its information and monitoring network and encouraging a broad partnership among governments, the voluntary sector, citizen action groups, and the business community.

Symposia such as this can concentrate scholarship on the health impact of rapid economic changes at this critical period in European history. They also provide the forum for discussion so necessary to making rational policy choices that are effective, equitable, and sustainable. We recognize that there is no "magic bullet" to prevent or even reduce the negative impact on people's health of many of the societal changes affecting the Region today. We also appreciate that different cultural and social traditions among the 50 Member States of the Region will inevitably call for different solutions. Indeed, this symposium brought out several of these variations on the theme. But that is precisely the point: we can agree on the common theme, where variations reflect the importance of the special circumstances of each country or subregion. A pan-European strategy for strengthening investments in health in all public policies begins with the kind of thoughtful, open dialogue this symposium so ably represents.

We trust that this report will stimulate debate among a wide circle of scholars, legislators, administrators, and social and health service practitioners. We challenge them to consider creative, even bold investments in health in public policies.

J.E. Asvall
WHO Regional Director for Europe

Vappu Taipale
Director-General
National Research and Development
Centre for Welfare and Health

Introduction
Lowell S. Levin
Laurie McMahon
Erio Ziglio

This is clearly not a propitious time to consolidate the vast, and disparate, literature on the social determinants of health. Given the rapid social changes engulfing the Region today, however, scholars and policy-makers must get together to gain a more up-to-date perspective on what we know, what gaps there are in our knowledge and what the priorities for health and social welfare research and intervention must be. There is a sense of urgency now to bring the issues into focus and to uncover the underlying values and principles that guide, or should guide, our policy choices, as we confront the crises that threaten the health and wellbeing of Europeans. The effects of political and economic changes in central and eastern Europe and the newly independent states of the former USSR are being felt throughout the Region. A pan-European perspective can and should lead to a sense of common cause with variations on the theme of solution, as these reflect particular national traditions and economic constraints.

An international symposium on the social determinants of health was therefore held in Helsinki, on 18–21 June 1993, and is expected to be the first in a series of symposia on the subject. The 30 participants, from Finland, Germany, Hungary, Sweden, the United Kingdom, the United States and Zambia (see Annex), met to present and discuss the papers contained in this publication.[a]

What is the value of this collection of papers on the relationship of economic and social change and health? Even a casual reading reveals several possibilities. The first is its contribution to calm and rationality. Each author carves out a specific aspect for clarification, which in some instances challenges conventional wisdom. A second impression is that the perceived "crisis" is really a continuing saga, with a vast amount of the baseline data needed to shape alternative scenarios and make alternative predictions still unavailable. An extraordinarily complex range of interacting variables emerges at both macro and micro levels.

[a] WHO gratefully acknowledges the financial support of the Finnish National Research and Development Centre for Welfare and Health for the printing of this publication.

1

Depending through which end of the telescope one looks, solutions to the social consequences of economic pressures focus on long-term structural strategies at the national level or short-term relief adjustments at the level of the individual. The papers assembled here help us appreciate both the necessity of having structural and programmatic solutions that complement each other and the inevitable dilemmas of providing long- and short-term solutions in the same development context.

A third contribution of this volume is to delineate the developmental circumstances of the so-called transitional states of central and eastern Europe and the welfare states of northern and western Europe. As one proceeds through the seven papers, it becomes clear that transitional is a term applicable to virtually all of Europe. In the case of central and eastern Europe, the transition is substantially more pervasive in all aspects of the political and economic fabric with a somewhat more pandemic effect on the health and welfare of the whole of society. For the northern and western countries of Europe, the economic transition is perhaps less evenly felt among subsets of the population. Several papers in this volume specify the groups at greatest health risk in the current economic downturn. The first-time unemployed are of special concern. The physical, social and mental health effects are shown as the poor get poorer and others join their ranks for the first time.

The impact of economic changes on morbidity and mortality in the Region is clearly of immediate concern. But even more ominous is the effect these changes have on the opportunities to promote health in more positive terms, to enhance the quality of life and the wellbeing of individuals, families and communities. The range of life choices and options for healthful lifestyles is reduced and physical and social environments are compromised. In effect, personal and social investments in health may drop to a lower priority on the political agenda. The struggle is now to seek ways and means of maintaining minimal service resources and structures to sustain the safety net.

In the face of deficits in national resources and, in some instances, an apparent national inability to resolve conflicting strategic options and take an effective leadership role, local communities are seeking solutions on their own initiative with their own resources. Local interest is growing in defining problems, setting priorities and taking local action where intersectoral collaboration is less encumbered by large bureaucracies and counterproductive jurisdictional disputes. Innovation emerges out of unity and a common cause. Apparently in some countries a belief is growing, perhaps out of frustration with the lack of effective central government action, that sustainable solutions require the responsible participation of all citizens and the strengthening of the community as a supportive environment.

The papers in Chapters 1 to 7 represent perspectives from economics, sociology, social welfare and health promotion, and from diverse cultural settings as well. The discussions that followed the presentation of each paper were analysed and synthesized by the London-based Office for Public Management in Chapter 8. Three major themes ran through the discussion:

1. the values and principles to be considered in formulating responsive policy;

2. the information and research required to understand the effects of rapid economic changes on health, welfare and employment; and

3. strategies for action.

The underlying concern for the northern European countries was made amply clear: how to preserve the social values of the welfare state while adjusting to the new budgetary stresses and their sequelae. The issue is how to design a social policy that maintains the principle of security for all, when clearly economic stressors are having an uneven demographic impact. The debate on targeted versus universal benefits showed that a substantial amount of new data is required on the health and social impact of rapid, economic change. Such data should account for a wide range of effects, both quantitative and qualitative, as well as the intensity and duration of those effects. Such data are needed at individual, family, community and national levels. A strong view was repeatedly put forward that community participation in the formulation of research on the impact of rapid economic change on people's health and welfare was essential to achieve a credible basis for effective policies. Of special interest was the insistence of the symposium participants that there be a stronger link between the health and social research communities and policy-making bodies. More "user friendly" research that communicates well with legislators and the public would help create the more rational and productive dialogue so essential in this period of competing, sometimes conflicting, social agendas.

The strategies for action suggested in the discussion of the papers provide a dramatic picture of the urgency of building multiple policy scenarios that identify the opportunities and costs associated with health investments in a wide range of public policy areas. These scenarios must also take account of health impact analyses that reflect the values and priorities of the population groups most affected by them. The symposium participants were in no doubt that the process of responding to the present social stressors on health must be a public process, rooted in sustainable community action, involving both public and private sectors, official and voluntary resources.

The clear intent of this publication is to help focus discussion of the impact of rapid social and economic change in the region on health and welfare. Health initiatives taken in the context of policy responses to the current circumstances of economic stress should be viewed as investments rather than expenditures. Creative investments in health should go beyond avoiding negative consequences to considering opportunities for building the capacity of individuals, communities and nations to advance the quality of life in general. Winston Churchill's admonition that "a crisis is a dangerous opportunity" seems most relevant to these times of rapid change and uncertainty.

The patterning of responses to unemployment: deprivation and adaptation

Eero Lahelma

In modern societies employment and unemployment are insep-arable institutions: unemployment could not exist without em-ployment. Unemployment, as the involuntary loss of paid work, implies that the unemployed are not workless; unemployed peo-ple certainly work, they do housework, some study, some work on a voluntary basis and some work in the informal economy. What unemployed people lack is a job and the remuneration entailed by it. Earning one's living in modern societies is inseparably interwoven with holding a job; no wonder therefore that unem-ployment is the main source of poverty in such societies.

The primary interest of this chapter is not the financial problems of unemployed people. Based on Freud's ideas of the significance of professional work, this chapter benefits, first, from Marie Jahoda's amazing scholarship on the significance of unem-ployment and employment over 60 years. It benefits, second, from the work of Peter Warr, who further developed Jahoda's ideas and put them to the test in an extensive research pro-gramme in the 1980s. These sources suggest that the significance of paid employment far exceeds that of financial remuneration only. Unemployed people face losses and difficulties, beyond poverty, that cannot be understood without reference to the significance of employment as a social institution.

The main argument of this chapter is that employment as an institution imposes on us a number of psychosocial require-ments. These requirements have become integral to modern life since the industrial revolution, and their strength lies in the fact that they are combined with as compelling a reason as earning one's living (1). As employment as an institution occupies such a central place in our lives economically, psychologically and socio-logically, we can expect large numbers of unemployed people to experience distress from their involuntary loss of employment. This is likely to continue as long as the institutional arrangements of modern societies endure.

Such "work societies" are predicted to end, but so far this holds true primarily in the sense that large groups of people remain involuntarily without a job, not in the sense that many people voluntarily stop looking for a job. In modern societies, examples of institutional arrangements for healthy middle-aged people to live outside paid employment are few indeed. The housewife role has been the main arrangement for living outside employment, although housewives are highly dependent on their husbands holding jobs. Further, this role is fading in countries such as Finland. The main trend has been for more and more women to take jobs, and there are pressures that ensure this development continues. Employment as an institution is not showing signs of weakening; on the contrary, new groups still continue to enter the labour market, the largest group being women.

The high significance of paid work in modern societies has been criticized for repressing people's own aspirations. "Useful unemployment" (2) and "dual" models of society (3) have been proposed to abolish the current institutions of employment and unemployment. These alternatives must be regarded as utopian; they have little to say when unemployment is examined as a "public issue" or as a "personal trouble" (4). My aim is not to undermine the critique of the social organization of employment and unemployment in modern societies. Nevertheless, we cannot ignore Jahoda's conclusions that:

> the needs met by employment are probably deeper and more enduring than the institutional arrangements to which we have become accustomed as satisfying them,

and that:

> these institutional arrangements are so intricately interwoven with the very nature of modern societies that they are likely to endure for a long time, certainly longer than it makes sense to look ahead (1).

It follows that the least that a "work society" can give the unemployed is financial compensation. But it also follows that unemployed people have needs that cannot be met by money alone; even sufficient compensation cannot prevent all the distress experienced by unemployed people. The aim of this chapter is, first, to understand the deprivation associated with unemployment through the significance of employment; second, to specify the patterning of this deprivation; third, to give an overview of current evidence on the patterning of deprivation among the unemployed, in terms of their mental and other dimensions of health; and, finally, to discuss the relevance of deprivation and adaptation among the unemployed with regard to health and welfare policies.

The pioneering work

In his essay *Civilization and its discontents*, Freud *(5)* strongly emphasizes professional work, or what we now call employment or paid work, in writing that:

> no other technique for the conduct of life attaches the individual so firmly to reality as laying emphasis on work; for his work at least gives him a secure place in a portion of reality, in the human community.

In the conduct of our lives, a reality principle allows us to avoid suffering from the external world. The best way of continuously testing our ties with reality is to engage in professional work in the community. There are other ways of striving for happiness and avoiding suffering, such as intoxication and religion, but they are far inferior as they entail turning away from the external world and relying on illusions *(5)*.

From Freud's viewpoint, paid work appears to have a broad significance ranging from the normative social order to personal identity. Above all, joining the community and engaging in paid work is psychologically a most economical way of pursuing happiness and avoiding suffering. The ties with our external environment provided by paid work also prevent us from becoming overwhelmed with fantasy and emotion *(6)*. Nevertheless, difficult social problems arise because "as a path to happiness, work is not highly prized by men" *(5)*.

Freud complains that he cannot discuss the significance of paid work adequately in that context. Fortunately, other scholars have continued this discussion. Without them, our understanding of the significance of employment and unemployment would be much more limited than it now is.

All research on the consequences of unemployment must pay tribute to the pioneering work of Jahoda and her colleagues, which started in the small village of Marienthal outside Vienna in 1931. As Fryer *(7)* noted recently, the Marienthal study by Jahoda, Lazarsfeld & Zeisel *(8)* "was to dominate research on unemployment and mental health for the next 60 years and probably beyond". Jahoda and her colleagues were not in fact the first to take up unemployment as a psychosocial and health problem. As they noted, Rowntree & Lasker's *Unemployment. A social study (9)* on unemployed people in York was the "first systematic sociographic study of unemployment" *(8)*. Rowntree & Lasker's interests were primarily poverty and the causes of unemployment, however, while Jahoda and her colleagues were interested in the mental state and response to unemployment. What makes the work of Jahoda and her colleagues so important is the thematization of unemployment as a deprivational experience, and the subsequent attempts to understand the nature of this deprivation among unemployed people.

Patterns of deprivation

This examination of the consequences of unemployment begins by emphasizing the significance of employment as a dominant social institution and the losses and suffering that follow exclusion from employment. In addition to this deprivation approach to the consequences of unemployment, Fryer proposes an alternative agency or pro-activity approach *(7,10)*. The agency approach concentrates on the activity and outlook of the unemployed, and the restrictions of activities faced by the unemployed, for example, due to poverty. The agency approach helps us understand differences in the responses of unemployed individuals; this approach emphasizes psychological considerations, such as the expectations for the future of unemployed individuals, and restrictions (usually economic) to these expectations.

The deprivation approach emphasizes the sociological consideration of employment as a social institution and allows a broad examination of the consequences of job loss *(11)*. This approach is justified if our aim is a general understanding of the response to joblessness. According to the deprivation approach to unemployment *(8)*, individual and family responses to unemployment can assume three or four adaptation types: the *resigned* category is the most common attitude; *broken* attitudes occur in individuals and families who are *in despair* or *apathetic*; in contrast to these more or less negative attitudes, a minority show an *unbroken* attitude. Although the main interest is in the negative or deprivational response to unemployment, neutral and positive responses exist as well. The fact that some unemployed people are mentally healthy reminds us that unemployment does not have to lead to mental problems *(7)*. This is an important point, as the consequences of the wave of mass unemployment since the 1970s have often been interpreted in a dramatic and deterministic way, particularly by the public and in the media *(12–14)*. Similarly, the results of research on deprived subgroups in the 1930s, suggesting that "unemployment is a profoundly corrosive experience, undermining personality and atrophying work capacities" *(15)*, could be applied to the present day.

Summarizing research at the end of the 1930s, Eisenberg & Lazarsfeld *(16)* formed a typology. Rather than showing alternative types of adaptation to unemployment, this suggested dynamic stages in the response to unemployment. The typology included the following four stages: unemployment causes an initial *shock*; this is followed by job seeking and *optimism*; lack of success leads to *pessimism*; the final stage involves a mental decline and *fatalism*. Taken literally and generalized to all unemployed people, this developmental view of the response to unemployment could lead to even more serious misinterpretations than does the use of the adaptation types. Studies and views of unemployment that postulated deterministic stages of deprivation and attributed these equally to all unemployed people gave an extremely pessimistic view of unemployment and contributed little to the understanding of unemployment and its consequences. A closer examination disclosed these misinterpretations; this encouraged a re-thinking of unemployment as a deprivational experience. Attention was drawn instead to the subjective and social conditions associated with unemployment (10,17,18). This resulted in emphasis being placed on the social construction of unemployment and the distress associated with it (7,19).

When Jahoda (1,20) returned to problems of employment and unemployment in the early 1980s, she defined the patterning of deprivation to improve our understanding of the significance of employment *and* unemployment. Employment as a social institution has manifest as well as latent consequences. Earning one's living is an intended and manifest consequence of employment. Additionally, employment imposes on the vast majority of employees a number of latent categories of experience, which follow from the structure of the institution of employment in modern societies. Thus, employment unintentionally influences our life in five ways: it imposes a daily *time structure*; it provides *social contacts* outside the family; it unites individual and collective *purposes*; it is a source of *status* and *identity*; and finally it is a source of *regularity* and being controlled. Jahoda concludes that deprivation among the unemployed occurs because these latent consequences of employment have become a requirement of modern life.

Warr (6) has developed Jahoda's ideas into a more detailed model for use in the study of unemployment and employment. This model contains nine environmental features: opportunity for control, opportunity for skill use, externally generated goals, variety, environmental clarity, availability of money, physical security, opportunity for interpersonal contact, and valued social position. The influence of these environmental features is similar to the effect of vitamins on physical health. The intake of vitamins, such as C and E, up to a certain level is important for physical health, but not beyond that level. Similarly, the absence of important environmental features is harmful to mental health, while their presence beyond a certain level does not yield any further benefit. The intake of some other vitamins, such as A and D, can even be harmful in very large quantities. Similarly, some features that contribute to mental health in moderate quantities may be harmful in very large quantities. For example, poverty is likely to have an adverse impact on mental health. Money is a remedy, although we cannot expect mental health to continue improving as more money is available. An excess of money, on the other hand, is unlikely to harm mental health. To take another example, to be able to control one's own work is beneficial to a certain extent, but excessive difficult decision-making may be harmful to mental health.

Warr's vitamin model has no context, but it has been strongly influenced by his research on unemployment. Job loss is likely to be followed by severe restrictions of the scope of the nine environmental features. The vitamin model therefore predicts, in a more detailed way than Jahoda's categories, that unemployment is likely to contribute to poor mental health.

The key message of Jahoda's five categories of experience or Warr's nine environmental features is not that they succeed in showing the exact consequences of employment and unemployment. Their advantage is primarily that they show, first, the importance of the institution of employment for modern life and, second, what kind of latent losses can follow from unemployment beyond the manifest losses of money.

Jahoda's & Warr's models are based on a reversal of Freud's statement that paid work provides people's strongest ties to reality, and indicate that these ties will tend to loosen in case of job loss. People's grip on reality requires continuous testing, and employment provides good opportunities for this, in the ways shown by Jahoda's five categories or Warr's nine environmental features. The unemployed have not lost their grip on reality but their opportunities are severely restricted. They know full well the financial hardships they face and their grip on reality is strong enough to know what they are missing, when they complain about boredom, being isolated or feeling depressed or anxious (1).

The above discussion does not allow us to judge exactly what kinds of patterns of mental deprivation are associated with unemployment. The deprivation due to unemployment depends on a number of conditions, and it is unlikely to follow a deterministic development. As unemployment and the suffering associated with it are ultimately socially constructed, the consequences of unemployment cannot be "logically entailed by the concept of unemployment" (21). The task of research is to show in a concrete way the patterning of deprivation and its conditions among the unemployed.

Health and deprivation

This section summarizes the evidence from research on deprivation in terms of health among the unemployed. Major emphasis is given to self-reported (nonpsychotic) mental health. Most studies examine this dimension of ill health, which is likely to be the immediate and dominant response to unemployment. Dimensions of health other than self-reported mental health fall largely outside the scope of this chapter. Nevertheless, two dimensions, that is, health-related lifestyles, particularly drinking behaviour, and mortality, will be considered briefly as they indicate divergent patterns of deprivation among the unemployed.

Mental health

The 1980s saw a revival of empirical research on the mental health of the unemployed. A number of large-scale surveys compared unemployed and employed people, using reliable and validated measures of nonpsychotic mental health, such as the General Health Questionnaire *(22)*. These studies show that unemployed people have much poorer mental health than their employed counterparts *(23–29)*.

Results from my own study among middle-aged Finnish industrial job seekers showed that about 50% of unemployed respondents, suffered from poor mental health compared with 20% or less of employed respondents, as measured by the General Health Questionnaire (Table 1). Percentages vary depending on the population studied and the measures used; the conclusion, however, is that mental health among unemployed and employed people shows large differences. Controlling for a number of other factors did not alter the main results. The association between unemployment and poor mental health is likely to be at its strongest in middle-aged people. It is also likely to be stronger for men than for women, but more research on women's response to unemployment is needed. The Finnish results agree broadly with results from comparable studies in several industrial countries.

Table 1. Percentage of unemployed and employed men and women
reporting poor mental health
(points 3–12 in the General Health Questionnaire 12-point score)

	Unemployed		Employed	
	Men (%)	Women (%)	Men (%)	Women (%)
First mailed questionnaire (1983)	54	37	18	17
Second mailed questionnaire (1984)	49	38	16	20

Note: 700 people answered the first mailed questionnaire and 698 people the second.

Source: Lahelma *(28,30)*.

To show an association between unemployment and mental health does not imply social causation, i.e. that unemployment is a cause of the poor mental health among the jobless. The association can just as well be explained by a drift hypothesis that implies that people with poor health are likely to become unemployed (7,11,31). Studies in which the basic level of mental health before becoming unemployed is known are rare, and social experimenting with unemployment is morally out of the question. In the course of longitudinal studies of unemployed people, however, re-employment takes place and this gives indirect evidence of the causal mechanisms behind the association of unemployment with poor mental health.

In the Finnish study, a positive improvement in mental health was associated with re-employment in a strong and exclusive way (28,30). A number of other studies have shown a similar effect: that finding a new job is followed by a rapid and substantial improvement in mental health (25, 27, 29,32–34). This evidence supports the social causation hypothesis: that the joblessness causes the poor mental health among the unemployed.

The experience of the unemployed can provide an overview of their mental health responses to unemployment and re-employment. From Warr's summary (6,35,36) and from other longitudinal studies referred to above, three instances of the impact of unemployment can be distinguished.

1. Typically, job loss tends to lead to an immediate impairment of mental health, although a small minority can gain in mental health after losing their job.

2. In the case of prolonged unemployment, mental health is likely to remain poor, although not necessarily to deteriorate further. In fact, a slight improvement in mental health can be expected over a long period of unemployment. According to Warr (6) this kind of adjustment to unemployment occurs about six months after job loss. A small minority of long-term unemployed people are likely to accumulate various problems with mental and physical health, the family and drinking, for example (37).

3. Re-employment is likely to lead to a rapid and substantial improvement in mental health.

Behind this overview, a number of circumstances can specify the individual responses to job loss and re-employment. People may respond differently to unemployment depending on the influence that Jahoda's latent categories of experience and Warr's nine environmental features had on their lives before they were unemployed.

First, the impact of age and gender has already been mentioned: middle-aged men are likely to respond particularly negatively to job loss. Second, a number of mechanisms can worsen the deterioration of mental health among the unemployed. These include financial worries, commitment to employment *(32)*, and inadequate social support *(25,27,38)*. Our picture of the complex of factors that interact with unemployment is rather sporadic, however. Third, particular subgroups of unemployed people can show divergent and even opposite responses to the general response. For example, highly educated or professional unemployed people have shown variable or neutral mental health responses to job loss *(39,40)*. More or less exceptional cases exist of positive responses to unemployment.

Most of the evidence shows that unemployment typically has a strong harmful impact on mental health. No clear routes such as poverty, however, can be found to mediate this mental deterioration among the unemployed. The adverse experience of job loss is often likely to be comprehensive, emphasizing the direct significance of loss of employment *per se*. This evidence supports Jahoda's & Warr's views on the strong psychological significance of the institution of employment.

Health-related lifestyle

Health-related lifestyles such as drinking are regarded, particularly by the public, as one of the mechanisms of deprivation among the unemployed. The debate about rising unemployment figures since the late 1970s stigmatized unemployed people as heavy drinkers, and sometimes characterized them as having a good time at "Costa del Dole". This preoccupation with the lifestyles of the unemployed has moralistic and political overtones.

In the examination of drinking behaviour and job loss, a distinction must be made between overall drinking levels and specific drinking problems. My study on industrial job-seekers in Finland *(41)* produced results that agreed with a number of other studies (Table 2). All these studies show that unemployed men and women are unlikely to drink more overall than their employed counterparts. If anything, they drink less, the main reason being their lack of money.

Being without a job is, however, likely to be associated with serious drinking problems among men, though not among women (Table 2). In other words, men report significantly more drinking-related health problems when unemployed than when employed.

In my study, the picture of overall drinking, as well as of drinking problems, remained the same when controlled for a number of other variables. Thus, unemployment is unlikely to increase overall drinking and accentuate in this way the deprivation of the jobless. Among unemployed men, however, a group of problem drinkers can be found, but unemployment is unlikely to have caused their drinking problems. On the contrary, their drinking behaviour probably stigmatized them and contributed to their unemployment.

Table 2. Percentage of unemployed and employed men and women
reporting drinking at least once a week; intoxication at least once a month;
and health problems due to drinking over the last 12 months

Reported behaviour	Men		Women	
	Unemployed (%)	Employed (%)	Unemployed (%)	Employed (%)
Drinking at least once a week				
First mailed questionnaire (1983)	58	53	22	27
Second mailed questionnaire (1984)	55	58	24	24
Intoxication at least once a month				
First mailed questionnaire (1983)	67	65	22	26
Second mailed questionnaire (1984)	65	60	23	22
Health problems due to drinking over 12 months				
First mailed questionnaire (1983)	32	20	10	9
Second mailed questionnaire (1984)	35	18	9	6

Note: Respondents to the first (and second) mailed questionnaire: 268 (155) unemployed men, 94 (207) employed men, 251 (121) unemployed women and 90 (220) employed women.

Source: Lahelma (40).

Thus, the drift hypothesis, rather than the social causation hypothesis, explains the association of men's drinking problems with their unemployment. A polarization hypothesis has also been proposed, suggesting that heavy drinkers may consume more alcohol when faced with the difficulties of unemployment, whereas moderate or light drinkers may reduce their consumption as part of a general cut-back in non-essential expenditure (6). In any case, available research suggests that unemployment does not contribute to excessive drinking or even to drinking-related problems, to any significant extent. The deprivation related to heavy drinking is more likely to be part of the selective processes in the labour market that tend to weed out heavy drinkers and the social closure experienced by stigmatized individuals and groups.

Few studies are available on the association of other health-related behaviours with unemployment. One recent study found that drinking and smoking were not associated with job loss, but gaining weight was *(42)*. Whether the association of health-related behaviours with unemployment follows similar or dissimilar patterns to drinking remains largely an open question *(43)*.

Mortality

In addition to lifestyles, the public has shown interest in the most extreme deprivation associated with unemployment: death. In a sense, death is the final stage of deprivation going far beyond fatalistic or apathetic attitudes. A deterministic model of deprivation would predict that unemployment, together with other unfavourable circumstances, is likely, at least in some cases, to end in premature death. According to some predictions, unemployment is likely to contribute to the premature death of large numbers of jobless people *(44)*. The public preoccupation with mortality and the unemployed is in part a wish to dramatize the consequences of unemployment.

Aggregate-level studies on unemployment and mortality *(44)* cannot establish an association at the individual level. Individual-level studies have shown that premature death is more common among unemployed than employed men. According to Martikainen's Finnish study *(45)*, mortality among unemployed men remained high even after controlling for a number of other variables. The unemployed were particularly prone to die suddenly, from causes of death such as accidents and violent acts, whereas associations between unemployment and gradual causes of death, such as cancer, and circulatory and other diseases, were much weaker or nonexistent. Furthermore, premature death became more common with prolonged unemployment. These results suggest social causation; in other words, that unemployment through direct or indirect mechanisms contributes to excess premature mortality among unemployed men.

Further studies by Valkonen & Martikainen *(46)* aimed at a more detailed analysis of the problem of causality. They have not confirmed, however, that unemployment causes the excess premature mortality of unemployed men. The possibility is hard to rule out that selection is due to factors that simultaneously contribute to both unemployment and premature death. The direction of causality remains an open question, and the drift hypothesis may explain the main part of the excess premature mortality found among Finnish unemployed men. The authors conclude that, "although unemployment has negative effects on the [mental] well-being of individuals, it is normally very exceptionally a catastrophe that kills".

Conclusion

This chapter has approached unemployment from a deprivation point of view. This viewpoint has been useful in 60 years of research on the consequences of unemployment. The general response of the unemployed has been specified, as have individual and group differences, to yield a picture of the deprivation among the unemployed. A major conclusion emerging from this research on health and unemployment is that various dimensions of health, such as mental health, health-related lifestyles and mortality, are likely to respond in a different way to job loss.

First, the consequences of unemployment for self-reported mental health are now well researched. Evidence from this research confirms that unemployment causes mental ill health, and re-employment is followed by improved mental health. Thus, large groups of unemployed people suffer mental deprivation owing to job loss. The mechanism of social causation is supposed to involve a rapid and substantial impairment of mental health in the case of job loss, and a rapid and substantial improvement of mental health in the case of re-employment. Prolonged unemployment is unlikely to continue to impair mental health, which reaches a plateau or improves slightly over a period of at least two years as adaptation occurs

In other words, the deprivational circumstances of unemployed people do not accumulate in a deterministic way that continuously aggravates their deprivation, leading finally to the total mental decline of large numbers of unemployed people. Fortunately, this is not the case; otherwise there would be hundreds of thousands of mentally ill people in need of hospitalization (36).

Second, the available evidence does not support the popular view that unemployment makes any major contribution to unhealthy lifestyles, such as heavy drinking. It is not, at least primarily, social causation but the drift hypothesis that is relevant here. Drinking behaviour labelled as deviant stigmatizes job seekers and prevents their re-employment. Lifestyle is unlikely to play an important role in the deprivation of the unemployed.

Third, research has established an association between premature mortality and unemployment. Although unemployment may contribute to the observed excess mortality, existing evidence does not show that unemployment *per se* is a major cause of the excess mortality. So far, convincing evidence of the direction of causality is missing, and the drift hypothesis is as plausible an explanation as the social causation hypothesis of the excess mortality among the unemployed (21). The same individual circumstances that entail a high risk of unemployment may also entail a high risk of morbidity and mortality, and these selective processes may produce the excess mortality observed among the unemployed. If this were the case, it would fit the pattern of mental deprivation among the unemployed: i.e. that, as a rule, mental deprivation due to job loss does not continue for ever and end in a total mental and physical decline.

Extreme responses to unemployment, negative as well as positive, are therefore likely to be uncommon and subject to special conditions. In Jahoda's words (47), excessive emphasis on the extreme responses to unemployment is a "wild exaggeration"; such responses may well occur in some cases, but not among the majority of the unemployed.

Discussion

If unemployment does not enhance unhealthy lifestyles and does not kill, but only causes mental distress, this pattern of deprivation among the unemployed can be considered reassuring. Or can it? My answer is, definitely not. It would be cynical to disregard the mental consequences of unemployment just because they "represent psychological burden and quality-of-life cost ... not expressed as mental hospital admissions" (31), because they are not dramatic enough to catch the public's attention (48) or because no serious political problems have arisen (49).

The end of this chapter aims to illuminate why ignoring the confirmed consequences for health of unemployment also excludes from policy considerations the benefits of paid work for people's life chances and wellbeing.

First, the mental health of the unemployed usually deteriorates in an undramatic way, with such symptoms as depression, anxiety and a sense of worthlessness. As the long-term unemployed adapt to their situation, however, their mental problems do not disappear. In the course of prolonged unemployment, mental health typically remains very poor, much worse than among comparable employed people (50). The symptoms of mental health that the unemployed report are, though, more obvious and more often recognized than a second type of injury.

Many long-term unemployed people show resigned adaptation. The term "resigned" refers to the adverse mechanisms lying behind this kind of adaptation. Without the consequences of employment, such as Jahoda's latent categories of experience and Warr's nine environmental features, the scope of unemployed people's lives is seriously restricted; as a result, "many long-term unemployed people have reduced their aspirations and turned in on themselves making them less of a problem to society" (48). Thus, because they adapt, the unemployed do not continue to suffer worsening deprivation. On the other hand, this very adaptation may entail deprivation of a more complex kind than can be judged from the state of their mental health alone.

Second, this chapter has used a negative concept of mental as well as other dimensions of health. Going beyond this to a positive concept of mental health draws attention not only to adjustment to the environment, but also to the potential for "psychological growth" and "self-realization" (6). Aspirations and involvement in the world are important keys to healthy living; "A slow decline into resigned adaptation which occurs with continuing unemployment is thus harmful in a fundamental way" (48).

Third, another point ignored in this chapter is an examination of the conditions inside the institution of employment, and the impact of unemployment on these conditions. Unemployment has been contrasted with employment all the way through this chapter. This has been a deliberate choice, but it is not intended to argue that all is well in the world of employment. Latent categories of experience (Jahoda) and environmental features (Warr) in employment can be very poor, so poor that they sometimes outweigh the consequences of unemployment (51). The case made here is that employment seldom has as adverse mental consequences as involuntary unemployment.

I started from Freud's viewpoint that paid work provides a person with his/her strongest ties to reality. I then followed Jahoda's & Warr's development of this viewpoint for a better understanding of the significance of employment for unemployment. This viewpoint leads to the conclusions, first, that work done in a paid job can be mentally beneficial even if it is not enjoyable and, second, that the loss of a job can be mentally damaging even in the case of a poor job (21). The aim was not, however, to argue that the conditions of employment are unimportant for health and wellbeing. It is just another unfortunate consequence of mass unemployment that the problems related to the conditions of employment tend to be pushed aside (1).

Finally, attention in this chapter has been devoted almost exclusively to ill health, mostly mental, as a response to unemployment. As seen in the Marienthal study 60 years ago, a minority of unemployed are unbroken (8). In my Finnish study, over half the unemployed responded neutrally or only slightly negatively about their mental health (28). Warr (36,52) calls "constructive adaptation" the response of those unemployed who take positive steps to develop interests and activities outside the labour market, and who engage in hobbies and voluntary work. This type of non-deprivational response to unemployment is uncommon, however, compared with the deprivational responses termed "resigned adaptation", which has been the main concern of this chapter.

Constructive adaptation needs to be examined side by side with resigned adaptation. Constructive responses can provide important experience for community interventions to help long-term unemployed people. Nevertheless, whether unemployed people can be encouraged to reduce their personal commitment to employment raises serious moral issues. These issues should be considered against the background that unemployment as a rule is an involuntary situation. Another important issue emerges directly from research: re-employment has proved to be the main remedy for the poor mental health of the unemployed.

References

1. JAHODA, M. *Employment and unemployment. A social-psychological analysis.* Cambridge, Cambridge University Press, 1982.
2. ILLICH, I. *The right to useful unemployment and its professional enemies.* London, Marion Boyars, 1978.
3. GORZ, A. *Paths to paradise. On the liberation from work.* New York, Pluto Press, 1985.
4. MILLS, C.W. *The sociological imagination.* New York, Oxford University Press, 1959.
5. FREUD, S. Civilization and its discontents. *In: The standard edition of the complete works of Sigmund Freud*, Vol. XXI. London, The Hogarth Press and the Institute of Psycho-Analysis, 1961.
6. WARR, P.B. *Work, unemployment and mental health.* Oxford, Oxford University Press, 1987.
7. FRYER, D. Editorial: introduction to "Marienthal and beyond". *Journal of occupational and organizational psychology*, **65**: 257–268 (1992).
8. JAHODA, M. ET AL. *Marienthal – the sociography of an unemployed community.* London, Tavistock, 1972.
9. ROWNTREE, B.S. & LASKER, B. *Unemployment. A social study.* London, Macmillan, 1911.
10. FRYER, D. & PAYNE, R. Being unemployed: a review of the literature on the psychological experience of unemployment. *In*: Cooper, C.L. & Robertson, I., ed. *International review of industrial and organizational psychology.* Chichester, Wiley, 1986.
11. JAHODA, M. Reflections on Marienthal and after. *Journal of occupational and organizational psychology*, **65**: 355–358 (1992).
12. SINFIELD, A. Unemployment in an unequal society. *In*: Showler, B. & Sinfield, A., ed. *The workless state.* Oxford, Martin Robertson, 1981.
13. DEACON, A. Unemployment and politics in Britain since 1945. *In*: Showler, B. & Sinfield, A., ed. *The workless state.* Oxford, Martin Robertson, 1981.
14. SIURALA, L. *Nuorisotyöttömyyden vaikutuksia – myytit ja todellisuus* [On the effects of youth unemployment – the myths

and the reality]. Helsinki, Ministry of Labour, 1982 (Työpolittisia tutkimuksia, No. 31).

15. HARRISON, R. The demoralizing effect of prolonged unemployment. *Employment gazette,* **84**: 330–349 (1976).

16. EISENBERG, P. & LAZARSFELD, P.F. The psychological effects of unemployment. *Psychological bulletin,* **35**: 358–390 (1938).

17. BONSS, W. ET AL. Das Ende der Belastungsdiskurses? Zur subjektiven und gesellschaftlichen Bedeutung der Arbeitslosigkeit. *In:* Bonss, W. & Heinze, R.G., ed. *Arbeitslosigkeit in der Arbeitsgesellschaft.* Frankfurt, Suhrkamp, 1984.

18. HARTLEY, J. & FRYER, D. The psychology of unemployment: a critical appraisal. *In:* Stephenson, G.M. & Davis, J.H., ed. *Progress in applied social psychology.* Chichester, Wiley, 1984, Vol. 2.

19. LAHELMA E. Paid employment, unemployment and mental well-being. *Psychiatria fennica,* **23**: 131–144 (1992).

20. JAHODA, M. & RUSH, H. *Work, employment and unemployment. An overview of ideas and research results in the social science literature.* Brighton, Science Policy Unit, University of Sussex, 1980.

21. WARR, P.B. Work, jobs and unemployment. *Bulletin of the British psychological society,* **36**: 305–311 (1983).

22. GOLDBERG, D.P. *The detection of psychiatric illness by questionnaire.* Oxford, Oxford University Press, 1972.

23. PAYNE, R. ET AL. Social class and psychological ill-health during unemployment. *Sociology of health and illness,* **5**: 152–174 (1984).

24. KESSLER, R.C. ET AL. Unemployment and health in a community sample. *Journal of health and social behaviour,* **28**: 51–59 (1987).

25. BOLTON, W. & OATLEY, K. A longitudinal study of social support and depression in unemployed men. *Psychological medicine,* **17**: 453–460 (1987).

26. BRENNA, A. ET AL. Unemployment and health: findings of a study in Sardinia. *In:* Schwefel, D. et al., ed. *Unemployment, social vulnerability and health in Europe.* Berlin, Springer-Verlag, 1987.

27. IVERSEN, L. & SABROE, S. Psychological well-being among unemployed and employed people after a company closedown: a longitudinal study. *Journal of social issues,* **44**: 141–152 (1988).

28. LAHELMA, E. Unemployment, re-employment and mental well-being. A panel survey of industrial jobseekers in Finland. *Scandinavian journal of social medicine,* Suppl. 43 (1989).

29. VERKLEIJ, H. Vulnerabilities of very long term unemployed in the Netherlands; results of a longitudinal survey. *In:* Starrin, B. et al., ed. *Unemployment, poverty and quality of working life.* Berlin, Edition Sigma, 1989.

30. LAHELMA, E. Unemployment and mental well-being: elaboration of the relationship. *International journal of health services*, **22**: 261–274 (1992).

31. DOOLEY, D. ET AL. Unemployment and alcohol disorder in 1910 and 1990: drift versus social causation. *Journal of occupational and organizational psychology*, **65**: 277–290 (1992).

32. WARR, P.B. & JACKSON, P. Factors influencing the psychological impact of prolonged unemployment and re-employment. *Psychological medicine*, **15**: 795–807 (1985).

33. ENSMINGER, M.E. & CELENTANO, D.D. Unemployment and psychiatric distress: social resources and coping. *Social science & medicine*, **27**: 239–247 (1988).

34. KESSLER, R.C. ET AL. Unemployment, reemployment, and emotional functioning in a community sample. *American sociological review*, **54**: 648–657 (1989).

35. WARR, P.B. Twelve questions about unemployment and health. *In*: Roberts, B. et al., ed. *New approaches to economic life*. Manchester, Manchester University Press, 1985.

36. WARR, P.B. The psychological impact of continuing unemployment: some longitudinal data and a general model. *In*: Schwefel, D. et al., ed. *Unemployment, social vulnerability and health in Europe*. Berlin, Springer-Verlag, 1987.

37. MANNILA, S. *Työhistoria ja syrjäytyminen* [Work career and social exclusion. A study of 61 Finnish job seekers with both health and labour market troubles]. Thesis, Department of Sociology, University of Helsinki, 1990.

38. SPRUIT, I.P. Vulnerability and unemployment– a process to ill-health and constraints on intervention strategies in the Netherlands. *In*: Starrin, B. et al., ed. *Unemployment, poverty and quality of working life*. Berlin, Edition Sigma, 1989.

39. MANNINEN, J. *Akateemiset työttömät työnhakijat* [Unemployed academic job seekers]. Thesis, Department of Education, University of Helsinki, 1992.

40. SCHAUFELI, W. Unemployment and psychological distress. Some results from two longitudinal studies among professional graduates and long-term unemployed professionals. *In*: Verhaar, C.H.A. & Jansma, L.G., ed. *On the mysteries of unemployment: causes, consequences and policies*. Dordrecht, Kluwer Academic Publishers, 1992.

41. LAHELMA, E. Unemployment – a drinking problem? *British Sociological Association Annual Conference, University of Essex, Colchester, 5–8 April 1993*. Durham, British Sociological Association (in press).

42. MORRIS, J.K. ET AL. Non-employment and changes in smoking, drinking, and body weight. *British medical journal*, **304**: 536–541 (1993).

43. KALIMO, R. & VUORI, J. *Työttömyys ja terveys. Tutkimuskatsaus* [Unemployment and health. A review]. Helsinki, Työterveyslaitos, 1992.

44. BRENNER, M.H. *Mental illness and the economy*. Cambridge, Harvard University Press, 1973.

45. MARTIKAINEN, P. Unemployment and mortality among Finnish men, 1981-5. *British medical journal*, **301**: 407-411 (1990).

46. VALKONEN, T. & MARTIKAINEN, P. The association of unemployment and mortality: causation or selection? *In*: Lopez, A. et al., ed. *Premature adult mortality in developed countries*. Oxford, Oxford University Press (in press).

47. JAHODA, M. Economic recession and mental health: some conceptual issues. *Journal of social issues*, **44**: 13-23 (1988).

48. WARR, P. This unhappy breed. *New society*, **10**: 16-18 (1987).

49. DE WITTE, H. On the social impact of youth unemployment: political radicalization and the decline of the work ethic? *In*: Verhaar, C.H.A. & Jansma, L.G., ed. *On the mysteries of unemployment: causes, consequences and policies*. Dordrecht, Kluwer Academic Publishers, 1992.

50. WARR, P.B. & JACKSON, P.R. Adapting to the unemployed role: a longitudinal investigation. *Social science & medicine*, **25**: 1219-1224 (1987).

51. GRAETZ, B. Health consequences of employment and unemployment: longitudinal evidence for young men and women. *Social science & medicine*, **36**: 715-724 (1993).

52. WARR, P.B. Individual and community adaption to unemployment. *In*: Starrin, B. et al., ed. *Unemployment, poverty and quality of working life*. Berlin, Edition Sigma, 1989.

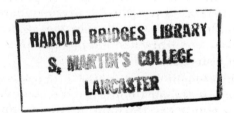

2

Effects of unemployment on mental wellbeing and health

Kaj Koskela
Heimo Viinamäki
Leo Niskanen
Osmo Kontula

In this chapter, we report on our study of the effects of unemployment and economic recession on mental wellbeing, using a group of personnel subject to job loss through factory closure plus a control group, and a randomly chosen population sample.

Background

Population studies usually compare unemployment figures with various official statistics on morbidity and mortality. Statistics are often interpreted after a certain delay as, in many illnesses, the effects of unemployment are only expected to be visible after several years. Such studies have focused on connections between unemployment and mortality in general, cardiovascular diseases, treatment in psychiatric hospitals, suicides and homicides.

A connection has been found between unemployment and the number of people seeking help for the first time for mental health problems [1]. In the United Kingdom, the number of admissions to psychiatric hospitals has been shown to increase as unemployment rises. The increase was particularly obvious among those who had previously received treatment for mental health problems [2]. On the other hand, the opposite results have also been obtained among people unemployed for more than 6 months [3].

Fryer & Payne [4] concluded that mental stress, negative emotions, unhappiness, dissatisfaction with life, and lack of enjoyment and positive emotions were more common among the unemployed than among people who had jobs. Follow-up studies showed that those who found a job during the follow-up period managed the above-mentioned factors better than those who remained unemployed.

Lahelma's questionnaire study on unemployed people in Finland (see Chapter 1) showed that unemployment posed a major threat to mental wellbeing *(5)*. Follow-up questionnaires were mailed in May 1983 and August 1984 to people who were unemployed in February 1983. Mental wellbeing had deteriorated in about half of those still unemployed, but in less than 20% of those who had found a job. This connection remained even after adjustment of background variables.

The effects of unemployment are perhaps most prolonged among young people just beginning their working life. Numerous studies show a connection between unemployment among young people and minor psychiatric disorders *(6)*. A British follow-up study showed that young people unable to obtain a job after finishing school had poorer mental health than employed people of the same age, although this difference was not visible while they were still at school *(7)*.

In the United Kingdom, a clear connection has been found between suicide, either attempted or successful, and unemployment. Unemployment does not, however, usually seem to lead to suicide directly; instead, mentally weaker people may end up unemployed more often than other people. Unemployment considerably exacerbates their mental health problems. If unemployment leads to poverty, the effect on mental health may be so great that the person commits, or at least attempts, suicide *(8)*.

The study

Against this background, the aim of our study was to investigate the effects of unemployment on mental wellbeing, using two study groups.

The study took place in Finland, where the number of unemployed increased sharply between 1990 (87 000 unemployed or 3.5%) and 1993 (470 000 unemployed or 19%). This was the fastest rise in any western country.

Subjects and methods
Study group 1
The first study group consisted of the entire personnel (211 people) of Finnforest, a wood processing factory in Hämeenlinna in southern Finland. All employees were given notice simultaneously in August 1991 as a result of rationalization procedures taken by the parent company. No significant reductions in the labour force had been made before this. The factory had been in business for 58 years.

The personnel (305 people) of a similar wood processing factory, Savon Sellu, in Kuopio in eastern Finland, acted as controls. The factory had been in business for 24 years. The average duration of employment was long and employee turnover low.

A questionnaire was mailed to the members of both groups in January 1992, and again in February 1992 to those who had not yet replied. The questionnaires were the same except that the one sent to Finnforest personnel had been extended to ask about the respondents' plans for coping with the future.

The questionnaires provided data on the respondents' age, sex, marital status, basic education, financial situation, social support and health. The subjects were also asked to describe their attitude towards the future.

Mental wellbeing was evaluated by means of three scales validated in earlier studies.

1. Psychological distress. The probability of minor psychiatric disorder (requiring psychological help) was assessed by means of the 12-item version of the General Health Questionnaire (GHQ) *(9,10)*. The items cover anxiety, depression, self-esteem and day-to-day difficulties and are scored from 0 to 12, with higher scores indicating greater ill health.

2. Depression. Depression was evaluated using a 13-item version of Beck's depression inventory (BDI) *(11)*. Responses were scored on a scale from 0 to 39, with higher scores indicating greater depression.

3. Psychosomatic reactivity. This was assessed subjectively by means of a 13-item list of psychosomatic symptoms (PS) compiled by Derogatis and colleagues *(12)*. Responses were scored on a scale from 0 to 52, with higher scores indicating a stronger tendency towards psychosomatic symptoms.

Study group 2

A population sample was interviewed by telephone. The interviews were carried out in conjunction with a study on manpower conducted by Statistics Finland. The interviews took place between 17 February and 1 March 1992.

Twice a year, a random sample of people aged 15–74 years and living permanently in Finland is taken from the central population register for the purposes of manpower studies. The addresses and other details about those in the sample are updated once a month using information obtained from the Population Register Centre.

The sample obtained in this way consists of about 2500 people. From the sample obtained in February, all those aged 18–74 years were included in the study. Before the interview they received a letter giving a brief account of the study.

The manpower study is usually carried out by telephone. Those study subjects whose telephone numbers cannot be found are interviewed in person. The study consisted of 90 interviews in person (5.7%) and 1499 telephone interviews (94.3%), giving a total of 1589 interviews (83.5% of the sample of 1930). The drop-out rate was thus 16.5%.

The respondents were divided into four groups: 652 employed people, 215 employed people who were afraid of losing their jobs, 51 employed people whose spouse was unemployed and 150 people who were unemployed. Retired people, students, those looking after their home and those doing military service were excluded from the study (a total of 862 people). As a result, unemployment closely concerned about 40% of the respondents: either they or people in their family were unemployed or they were afraid of losing their jobs.

Statistical analyses were carried out using the SPSS-X statistics package. The chi-squared test was applied to discrete variables, and the t-test, or Mann & Whitney's U-test, where appropriate, to continuous variables.

Results
Study group 1
Seventy-nine per cent of the study group and sixty-five per cent of the control group returned the questionnaire; 33 subjects in the study group were excluded from the analysis because they had already found a new job. Hence, the final size of the study group was 136 people. The mean age of the men in the study group was 44.3 ± 10.6 years and that of the women 45 ± 10.6 years (p = not significant). The mean age of the male controls was 43 ± 9.1 years and that of the female controls 41.7 ± 10.5 years (p = not significant). The proportion of men in the study group was 70% and in the control group 84%. The two groups were similar in terms of marital status and basic education.

The mental wellbeing of the subjects in the two groups is shown in Table 1, where the higher the score, the worse the mental state. The women in the study group (who were unemployed) were neither more depressed (BDI score) nor in greater need of psychological help (GHQ score) than the female controls (who were employed). Employed women showed more psychosomatic symptoms (PS score) ($p < 0.001$) than those who were unemployed. The men in the study group needed psychological help more often ($p < 0.001$) and were more depressed ($p < 0.01$) than the male controls (13).

Men of all ages in the study group needed more psychological help than the controls. Male controls aged 45–49 showed more psychosomatic symptoms than those who were unemployed (PS score 8.6 ± 1.1 versus 4.5 ± 2.0 ($p < 0.01$)). Men in the study group

Table 1. The mental wellbeing of the study group (unemployed)
and control group (employed)

Scale of measurement	Mean score (± standard error)			
	Study group		Control group	
	Men (N = 93)	Women (N = 43)	Men (N = 167)	Women (N = 31)
GHQ	3.7 ± 0.4[a]	2.8 ± 0.5	1.1 ± 0.2	2.3 ± 0.6
BDI	9.4 ± 1.1[b]	9.9 ± 1.6	5.8 ± 0.7	11.8 ± 2.4
PS	6.4 ± 0.8	6.4 ± 1.0[a]	7.6 ± 0.6	12.3 ± 1.3

[a] The difference between the scores of the study group and control group (of the same sex) is significant ($p < 0.001$), using Mann & Whitney's U-test.

[b] The difference between the scores of the study group and control group (of the same sex) is significant ($p < 0.01$), using Mann & Whitney's U-test.

aged 45–49 had poorer mental wellbeing than younger and older men (GHQ score 4.6 ± 1.1, BDI score 8.4 ± 2.3).

The mental wellbeing of men in both groups is shown in Table 2 in terms of their marital status. Single, divorced and widowed men in the study group suffered less from impaired mental wellbeing than married men. No similar tendency was observed in the controls. The married men in the study group needed more psychological help ($p < 0.001$) and were also more depressed ($p < 0.001$) than the controls.

The study group subjects were also asked to assess their ability to cope in the future. Unemployment and uncertainty about the future were associated with the greatest need for psychological help and the most severe depression. Those men who had confidence in the future coped better than the others in the study group (Table 3).

We also studied the effects of social support (14) and financial stress (15) on the mental wellbeing of men and women in the study group. The respondents assessed the level of their social support by answering the question: "Do you feel the people closest to you give you sufficient understanding and support in your problems?". The answers were assigned to a four-point scale. Two classes were formed: adequate and insufficient social support. Those who considered their social support insufficient needed more psychological help, had more psychosomatic symptoms and were more depressed than the others (Table 4).

Table 2. The mental wellbeing of the men of the study group (unemployed) and control group (employed) according to marital status

	Mean score (± standard error)					
Marital status	Study group (N = 93)			Control group (N = 167)		
	GHQ	BDI	PS	GHQ	BDI	PS
Unmarried	3.6 ± 0.9	7.9 ± 2.0	7.1 ± 1.8 (N = 18)	1.6 ± 0.6	7.5 ± 2.1	8.8 ± 1.8 (N = 20)
Married	3.9 ± 0.5[a]	10.2 ± 1.4[a]	6.6 ± 0.9 (N = 66)	0.9 ± 0.2	5.1 ± 0.7	7.3 ± 0.6 (N = 139)
Divorced/ widowed	2.1 ± 0.8	4.5 ± 2.6	2.3 ± 1.0[b] (N = 9)	3.3 ± 1.5	18.0 ± 6.1	8.4 ± 2.3 (N = 8)

[a] The difference between the scores of the study group and control group (of the same marital status) is significant (p < 0.001), using Mann & Whitney's U-test.

[b] The difference between the scores of the study group and control group (of the same marital status) is significant (p < 0.05), using Mann & Whitney's U-test.

Table 3. The mental wellbeing of the men of the study group (unemployed) and control group (employed) according to their expectations for the future

	Mean score (± standard error)					
Expectations for the future	Study group (N = 93)			Control group (N = 167)		
	GHQ	BDI	PS	GHQ	BDI	PS
Confident	1.5 ± 0.4[a]	3.7 ± 0.9	3.7 ± 0.7[a] (N = 53)	0.7 ± 0.2	3.4 ± 0.7	6.9 ± 0.7 (N = 99)
Uncertain	4.8 ± 0.5[b]	13.4 ± 1.6	8.3 ± 1.1 (N = 40)	1.8 ± 0.3	9.5 ± 1.3	8.7 ± 1.0 (N = 68)

[a] The difference between the scores of the study group and control group (with the same expectations for the future) is significant (p < 0.01), using Mann & Whitney's U-test.

[b] The difference between the scores of the study group and control group (with the same expectations for the future) is significant (p < 0.001), using Mann & Whitney's U-test.

The respondents also assessed their financial situation by means of a four-point scale. Two classes were formed: at least moderate, or poor financial status. A poor financial situation among the unemployed was associated with impaired mental wellbeing. Those in poor financial situations needed more psychological help, had more psychosomatic symptoms and were more depressed than the others (Table 5).

Table 4. The mental wellbeing of the study group
according to the social support they receive

Social support	Mean score (± standard error)		
	GHQ	BDI	PS
Adequate (N = 115)	3.0 ± 0.4[a]	7.8 ± 0.9[a]	5.4 ± 0.6[b]
Insufficient (N = 21)	6.5 ± 1.1	19.3 ± 2.6	11.5 ± 1.9

[a] $p < 0.001$, Mann & Whitney's U-test.
[b] $p < 0.01$, Mann & Whitney's U-test.

Table 5. The mental wellbeing of the study group
according to their financial situation

Financial situation	Mean score (± standard error)		
	GHQ	BDI	PS
At least moderate (N = 87)	2.7 ± 0.5[a]	7.9 ± 1.1[b]	5.3 ± 0.6
Poor (N = 49)	5.1 ± 0.6	12.1 ± 1.7	8.2 ± 1.2

[a] $p < 0.01$, Mann & Whitney's U-test.
[b] $p < 0.05$, Mann & Whitney's U-test.

Study group 2

In terms of social circumstances, the unemployed differed from the employed in that 35% lived alone or were single parents. Among the employed not afraid of losing their jobs, the corresponding figure was 20%. Living in a marriage or a marriage-like relationship was 15% more common among the employed than the unemployed. This difference was slightly exaggerated because the unemployed were on average somewhat younger than the employed. These findings are described elsewhere in detail (16).

Regular smoking was much more common among the unemployed (38%) than the employed not afraid of unemployment (21%). This difference was clear in all age groups. The groups did not differ from each other in terms of consumption of either beer or spirits. The unemployed drank wine far less often than the others. More unemployed than employed people reported having reduced their consumption of beer, wine and spirits over the past year.

Alcohol-related problems during the past year were slightly more common among the unemployed (6%) than people with jobs (2%). This may suggest that some unemployed people use alcohol as a means of coping.

The mental status of the unemployed was somewhat poorer than that of employed people not afraid of unemployment. The unemployed more often reported mental health problems, suicidal thoughts and diminished zest for life. In this respect, employed people who were afraid of losing their jobs were the most vulnerable group. These people seem very sensitive to changes in their environment. In many cases, their jobs really are at risk. This observation confirms the previous finding that the mere threat of unemployment or advance notice about it may impair mental health (Table 6).

None of the unemployed had sought help for psychiatric symptoms or problems in personal relationships over the previous six months. Just over 1% of those with jobs had received this type of therapy.

In terms of their own assessment of the future, the use of hypnotics or sedatives and perceived symptoms of mental ill health, the unemployed seemed to be in a slightly poorer situation than those who had jobs and were not afraid of unemployment. The unemployed had a very pessimistic view of the future. Again, those who had jobs but were afraid of losing them had problems as often as the unemployed. Mental health problems and the use of sedatives were most common among people whose spouses were unemployed. This is mainly because this group contained more wives of unemployed men than husbands of

Table 6. Incidence of mental health problems, suicidal thoughts and diminished zest for life in relation to employment status

Employment status	Percentage of people reporting:		
	mental health problems	suicidal thoughts	diminished zest for life
Employed (N = 652)	16.6	1.7	7.7
Afraid of unemployment (N = 215)	29.3	4.2	19.6
Unemployed spouse (N = 51)	35.3	2.0	8.0
Unemployed (N = 150)	23.3	2.7	13.3

unemployed women. Women generally use sedatives and report mental health problems more often than men. These problems are aggravated if the husband is unemployed (Table 7).

The use of sedatives was more common among middle-aged unemployed people than employed people of the same age. There were more first-time users in this age group than in the other groups. Excluding employment-related relationships, there were no differences between the unemployed and the employed in the social support they received.

In the present study, the unemployed differed from those who were unafraid of losing their jobs in having slightly poorer health, as judged both by their own assessment of their health status and by the illnesses diagnosed by a physician. The differences were fairly small, however. The spouses of unemployed people and those who were afraid of losing their jobs had illnesses diagnosed by a physician more often than the unemployed (Table 8).

The difference in health was most obvious among middle-aged people: the incidence of ill health was four percentage points higher among the unemployed than the employed.

Ill health was most common among middle-aged people who were afraid of losing their jobs. They seemed more sensitive than others to environmental changes threatening their livelihood.

No differences were found between the unemployed and those with jobs as far as the use of prescribed medication was concerned. On the other hand, a higher percentage (12%) of the unemployed reported having used more prescribed medication

Table 7. Incidence of uncertainty about the future,
use of hypnotics or sedatives and mental ill health
in relation to employment status

Employment status	Percentage of people reporting:		
	uncertainty about future	use of hypnotics or sedatives	mental ill health
Employed (N = 652)	3.7	6.8	34.6
Afraid of unemployment (N = 215)	15.4	5.6	43.8
Unemployed spouse (N = 51)	8.0	11.8	32.7
Unemployed (N = 150)	15.3	8.7	39.5

27. ELDER, G.H.J. & ROCKWELL, R.C. Economic depression and postwar opportunity in men's lives: a study of life patterns and health. *Research in community and mental health*, **1**: 249–303 (1979).

28. PLATT, S. Unemployment and suicidal behaviour: a review of the literature. *Social science & medicine*, **19**: 93–115 (1984).

29. HAWTON, K. & ROSE, N. Unemployment and attempted suicide among men in Oxford. *Health trends*, **18**: 29–32 (1986).

30. PLATT, S. & KREITMAN, N. Long-term trends in parasuicide and unemployment in Edinburgh, 1968–87. *Social psychiatry and psychiatric epidemiology*, **25**: 56–61 (1990).

31. CROMBIE, I.K. Trends in suicide and unemployment in Scotland, 1976–86. *British medical journal*, **298**: 782–784 (1989).

32. PRITCHARD, C. Is there a link between suicide in young men and unemployment? A comparison of the UK with other European Community countries. *British journal of psychiatry*, **160**: 750–756 (1992).

33. SMART, R.G. & MURRAY, G.F. Drug abuse and affluence in five countries: a study of economic and health conditions, 1960–1975. *Drug and alcohol dependence*, **11**: 297–307 (1983).

34. SMITH, R. "Without work all life goes rotten". *British medical journal*, **305**: 972 (1992).

3

Income distribution, income change and health: on the importance of absolute and relative income for health status in Sweden

Olle Lundberg
Johan Fritzell

Background

In this chapter, we describe our study[a] of the relative importance of the absolute and relative dimensions of income for people's health. We studied the physical and psychological health of a sample of people 35–64 years old, taken from a national population sample, in relation to the absolute and relative changes in their income between 1980 and 1990.

That material circumstances and wealth are closely linked with illness and health has been documented and proven on innumerable occasions. One well known example of this is in the writings of Engels in *The condition of the working class in England* *(1)*, and an even earlier example can be found in Sweden *(2)*. The notion of material deprivation as the most forceful factor behind illness and mortality among large segments of the population also influenced the social reform movement in Europe during the 1840s *(3)*. More recently, however, the focus has shifted towards other factors, predominantly health-related behaviour such as smoking and diet, or social relations such as social networks and social support. This shift in focus is probably rooted in the vast improvements in affluence that have taken place over the last 100 years.

---

[a] This study was supported by the Swedish Council for Social Research.

Despite increasing prosperity and the rise in standards of living during the past century, income or economic resources may still be important for health. Differences in economic resources are likely to be related to differences in illness and mortality between groups in countries and between countries. The importance of economic resources will probably also become more visible during periods of economic recession.

Although the main interest of many researchers in public health has been the social rather than the economic factors behind illness, economic aspects have not been omitted totally from the analyses. In three important areas, research and debate have centred on the association between economic resources and health. These areas are childhood conditions and later adult health, class differences in health, and income distribution and health.

Childhood conditions and adult health

Over the past 15 years, a number of studies have presented data that suggest that living conditions during childhood, or even the living conditions of the pregnant woman, are important for illness and mortality in later adult life. Forsdahl (4,5) and Barker & Osmond (6,7) have published ecological data, where differences in infant mortality between geographical areas have been shown to correlate with variations in cardiovascular mortality at a later stage. Further, from individual data, a relationship has been established between childhood conditions (such as birth weight, childhood health status or socioeconomic position of the child's family) and adult mortality (8–12). A recent study demonstrated that economic hardship during childhood (up to the age of 16) was related to adult health (Table 1). The study looked at 4216 people aged 30–75 years in 1981, and controlled for sex, age and the social class of the father. It showed that economic hardship during childhood is a predictor of adult illness, even when other childhood problems, as well as age, sex and the social class of the father, are controlled for. Dissension in the family is a stronger predictor, however, indicating that economic deprivation is but one factor operating here.

Even if the criticism of the studies referred to above is taken into consideration (14–16), there is strong support for the existence of a relationship between childhood conditions and adult illness and mortality, although economic deprivation is only one of several possible factors.

The suggested mechanism behind this relationship is that economic deprivation during critical periods of fetal and/or childhood development affects physiology and metabolism in a way that increases the risk of cardiovascular disease (17). This has been labelled the biological imprint hypothesis (13). An alternative hypothesis is that economic deprivation in childhood is associated with a number of unfavourable living conditions

Table 1. Odds ratios for certain forms of ill health in 1981
or mortality in 1981–1984, for adults exposed to various
childhood conditions compared with adults who were not thus exposed

Measure of ill health	Childhood conditions			
	Economic hardship	Large family	Broken family	Dissension in family
General physical ill health	1.26 (0.0095)	1.20 (0.0199)	1.26 (0.0273)	1.73 (0.0001)
Aches and pains	1.43 (0.0001)	1.12 (0.1745)	1.27 (0.0381)	1.76 (0.0001)
Circulatory illness	1.10 (0.4426)	1.27 (0.0446)	1.70 (0.0005)	1.81 (0.0010)
Mental illness	1.50 (0.0008)	1.35 (0.0093)	1.56 (0.0017)	2.14 (0.0000)
Mortality (spring 1981–end 1984)	1.10 (0.5586)	1.10 (0.5320)	1.32 (0.1723)	1.52 (0.0628)

Note: p-values in parentheses.

Source: Lundberg (13).

during life, and that illness in adulthood is a result of the joint effects of these conditions – the unhealthy life career hypothesis (13). Economic factors have only an indirect role in both these hypotheses, namely as markers for health-damaging factors such as poor nutrition or unsafe working conditions. Finally, only the absolute dimension of income has been assumed to be at work here. Thus differences in the level of income lead to differences in nutrition and so on during infancy or childhood, which in turn have health consequences later on in life.

Causes of class inequalities in health

The debate on the causes of the inequalities in illness and mortality between social classes includes, although not always explicitly, the level of economic resources as a possible explanatory factor. Particularly in the British literature, where social class is taken as a proxy indicator of poverty and wealth, class differences in health are often seen as the result of economic deprivation. Again, the absolute level of income is usually the focus, as manifested in car ownership or public housing (18,19). In the classic Black report, however, relative deprivation was also taken as an important factor leading to class differences in illness and mortality (20). In this respect, the Black report closely follows the earlier works of Peter Townsend (21), where he has argued for a relative definition of poverty.

Although many possible factors have been suggested as causes of the persistent class differences in health, few studies have actually tried to test their relative importance. One exception is a study carried out by Lundberg *(22)* on a representative sample of 6174 people from the Swedish population aged 15–75 years in 1981. This study considered childhood conditions, economic resources, physical working conditions, the mental strain of the workplace, social support and health-related behaviour as factors that may contribute to class inequalities in health. All these factors were shown to be related to illness, as well as to class position. The relative contribution of the factors to class differences in health was assessed by adding each factor in a logit regression model including class, age and sex, first one by one, and then as the last variable in a full model. Hence, those factors that were associated with a large decrease in class differences when included in the model contribute most to class differences.

Fig. 1 shows that physical working conditions were the most important set of factors behind class differences in illness, followed by health-related behaviour (tobacco and alcohol consumption) and economic hardship during childhood. Differences in economic resources in adult life, on the other hand, do not seem to produce health inequalities between social classes in Sweden.

Fig. 1. Percentage change in class differences in physical illness, when factors are added to the model as the only factor (gross change) or as the last factor (net change)

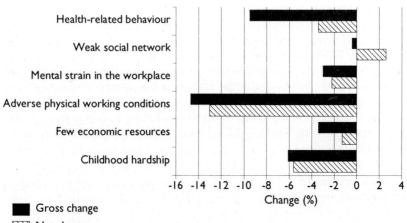

Gross change
Net change

Source: Lundberg *(22)*.

This implies that, in Sweden at least, income or economic resources are of no great importance for class differences in health. On the other hand, since income differences, both in general and between classes, are smaller in Sweden than in most other countries, these results may not enable one to draw conclusions about other countries. This leads us to the third area of research where income has been related to health.

Income, income distribution and health

Class differences in health status within countries are hardly surprising. Nor is the inverse correlation between mortality and gross national product per head in many countries around the world. This correlation, however, is far from perfect. Several countries are very poor by economic standards but have still managed to increase their life expectancy dramatically (23). Furthermore, this correlation no longer seems to hold among the richer countries. Instead, one of the most astonishing and puzzling results of recent social science research is the impact of income inequality on classical health measurements such as infant mortality and life expectancy.

Thus, ample evidence now suggests that in industrialized countries further increases in gross national product will not greatly improve life expectancy or various measures of health status. Instead, this research implies that a dampening of income differentials will be the most effective way of improving people's health. Thus, le Grand (24), Rodgers (25), Wennemo (26) and Wilkinson (27,28) all report that in rich countries the impact of gross domestic product per head is negligible on cross-national variations in different aggregate measures of morbidity and mortality.

Instead, income inequality seems to be strongly correlated with mortality. Thus, countries with little inequality and a low incidence of relative poverty also tend to have lower infant mortality rates and higher life expectancy. Hence, since the marginal return of income on health probably diminishes as one moves up the income scale, decreasing income differentials should improve the average health status and the average life expectancy of a country. Wilkinson follows this line of thought even further by arguing that, if income is redistributed from the rich to the poor, not only is the health of the poor improved but in fact: "health might improve at both extremes simultaneously" (27).

The reason for this seemingly odd argument is that he claims to find support for a reverse-J relationship between income and health in a large cross-sectional study by Blaxter (18). Thus, the percentage of ill people decreases as income increases, but becomes larger again in the highest income groups. Even though such a relationship in a cross-sectional data set is not a proper test

Table 2. The relative income change (R) resulting from different combinations of absolute changes in mean and individual income levels

Absolute change in mean income level \ Absolute change in individual income level	+	0	–
+	1 R +/0/–	2 R –	3 R –
0	4 R +	5 R 0	6 R –
–	7 R +	8 R +	9 R +/0/–

In our study, where we compared the income level in 1980 with that of 1990, the median income increased in real terms (net of inflation). Among the panel sample we selected, it increased by SKr 15 250 (US $1906 in 1994) per annum. This means that only the combinations in the top row of Table 2 are available in our data. To show the possible combinations of absolute and relative changes in individual income level, given this constraint, we can make a new matrix based purely on the individual level (Table 3).

From Table 2, it follows that four combinations in Table 3 are logically impossible. These are shaded. Of the remaining combinations, cell 1 and 9 represent those cases where the absolute change, negative or positive, is combined with a similar relative change. In these combinations, therefore, one cannot really disentangle the relative from the absolute effects of income on health. If, however, the health of those in cell 1 is worse than the health of those in cells 4 or 7, then the absolute level of income is important for health status. Similarly, the relative dimension is important if those in cell 9 have better health than those in cells 7 or 8.

Table 3. Possible combinations of absolute and relative changes
in individual income during the 1980s

Absolute change \ Relative change	−	0	+
−		1 //// 2 ////	3 ////
0		4 //// 5 ////	6 ////
+		7	8	9

The study

The effects of income on health need closer analysis, especially the relative importance of the absolute versus the relative dimension of income. For such an analysis to be meaningful, a relationship between income and health must, of course, exist in the first place. Since income changes may follow from ill health, the analysis of absolute versus relative income changes and health must take this into account. Furthermore, income changes, both absolute and relative, may have different impacts on health according to the initial income level. Our study, therefore, focused on the following questions.

1. Is health related to income in Sweden?

2. Are absolute and relative income changes related to health?

3. If income changes are related to health, do these relationships hold when the initial income level and initial health status are controlled for?

Data

The data source we used stems from the Swedish Level of Living Survey. These surveys have been conducted four times (in 1968, 1974, 1981 and 1991) using a panel design. In each one, around 6000 individuals, forming a random sample of the Swedish population aged 15–75 years, were interviewed about their general living conditions, including a broad section on health status. (For a more elaborate presentation of the data set, see Erikson & Åberg *(33)*.) In addition to the information gleaned from the interviews, a large number of variables, mainly relating to incomes, were collected from different administrative registers. We used data from the 1981 and 1991 surveys and thus included only those responding to both surveys. We further restricted our sample to those aged 35–64 years in 1991, and excluded housewives and the self-employed. The rationale for these exclusions is that housewives have no earnings and that income is a fairly poor measure of economic status among the self-employed. The characteristics of our sample are described in Table 4.

Independent variables

Age was used as a control variable, with three categories (35–44 years, 45–54 years and 55–64 years in 1991). Since both income and health differ systematically between men and women, all analyses were performed for each sex separately.

Income was measured as the annual individual taxable income in 1980 and 1990. Almost all earnings-related benefits in Sweden are taxable; the income measure thus includes sick pay, unemployment benefits, etc. From these data, two income measures were constructed, one reflecting the absolute level of income, and one the mobility within the income distribution.

The first of these measures was derived by forming ten and five income groups, separated by the decile and quintile values, respectively. These interdecile and interquintile groups then represented different income segments of the population, where

Table 4. Number of people in study sample,
by age group and sex

Age group (years)	Men	Women	Total
35–44	364	350	714
45–54	368	332	700
55–64	225	235	460
Total	957	917	1874

the tenth interdecile group was the 10% of the population with the largest incomes, and the first interquintile group was the 20% with the lowest incomes. The interdecile grouping was used for the analysis of absolute income and health, as well as for constructing the measure of absolute and relative change in income. The interquintile grouping was used as a control variable in the multivariate analyses of the importance of income changes. Both the interdecile and the interquintile groups were constructed on the basis of men and women taken together.

The second indicator was designed to capture different types of income change between 1980 and 1990, i.e. different types of mobility between and stability within the interdecile groups. We have discussed the theoretical rationale behind this indicator (Tables 2 and 3). To construct a measure that separates absolute and relative changes, following the principles in Table 3, we first had to construct measures of relative and absolute change that have the values drop, remain stable and increase.

For the relative dimension, we used mobility in the income distribution, as indicated by change in interdecile group. Hence, people who were in a lower interdecile group in 1990 than in 1980 had experienced a relative drop in income.

This means, however, that people who experienced only a minor drop or increase in relative income may have remained within the interdecile group, and therefore no change was registered. This could partly have been solved by dividing the income distribution into smaller groups, but that would have increased the risk of including very small and insignificant changes. Thus, small changes in incomes close to the decile values would be more likely to entail a change of interdecile group. That is also a problem, of course, when working with 10% groups, as we did. A solution would have been to rule out mobility to the adjacent interdecile group as a change in position, but that would have increased the problem of some changes being hidden. In sum then, we are aware of the problems with our approach, but felt that other possible solutions would have caused just as many problems.

For the absolute dimension, the problem was to identify a group with a stable income. Strictly speaking, one should count only those with exactly the same yearly income in both 1980 and 1990 (net of inflation) as having a stable income. A more sensible approach was to choose an interval around this point of no absolute change, and to regard those within this range as having stable incomes. Thus income decreases or increases no greater than half the median change in income in our sample were defined as a stable absolute income. This meant that if:

1990 income = 1980 income $\pm$ SKr 7625 (US $990 in 1994)

then the income level was regarded as stable. If the level of income decreased by more than SKr 7625, a drop in absolute income had occurred, and if the yearly income increased by more than SKr 7625, then an absolute increase had taken place.

By cross-tabulating these two indicators, we constructed an empirical representation of Table 3, as Table 5.

Table 5 shows that our definitions of relative and absolute income changes led to 57 people ending up in cells 2 and 5. This, however, was logically impossible according to the more theoretically strict definition of absolute and relative change used in Table 2. Therefore, and since these cases were so few, we excluded them from the analyses.

The remaining combinations created a four-category variable. The first category comprised those with both absolute and relative increases in income between 1980 and 1990 (cell 9). The second was formed by those who experienced an absolute increase, but not a relative increase (cells 7 and 8). We would have preferred to count the most contradictory category in cell 7 as a category of its own, but the small number of cases in that cell made this impossible. The third category contained those who dropped in relative but not in absolute terms (cell 4), and the last category included those who experienced a drop both absolutely and relatively (cell 1). These categories are summarized in Table 6.

Table 5. Number of each possible combination of absolute and relative changes in individual income during the 1980s

Absolute change \ Relative change	−	0	+
−	1 360	2 (19)	3
0	4 249	5 (38)	6
+	7 90	8 429	9 751

Table 6. Construction of categories of the indicator
on income change, their labels and number of people

Category	Cell number	Label	Number of people
Absolute and relative increase	9	A+R+	751
Absolute increase, relative stable or drop	7+8	A+R0/–	519
Absolute stable, relative drop	4	A0R–	249
Absolute and relative drop	1	A–R–	360

Dependent variables

Two health indicators were included in this study, one covering
physical illness and one psychological distress. These indicators
were measured in the same way for the 1981 and 1991 samples.
The basis for both these measures was the question, "Have you in
the last 12 months had any of the following illnesses or ailments?", followed by a list of 50 items covering the most common
illnesses and ailments. To each item, the respondent was asked to
answer "No", "Yes, mild" or "Yes, severe".

To form the indicator of psychological distress, an additive
index is computed from the items "general tiredness", "insom-
nia", "nervous trouble (anxiety, uneasiness, anguish)", "depression", "deep dejection" and "over-exertion". The answer "No" is
given 0 points, "Yes, mild" is given 1 point and "Yes, severe" 3
points. If the respondent scores 3 points or more on this index, *or*
has reported having "mental illness", he or she is given the code
"yes" on the psychological distress indicator.

The indicator of physical illness includes all the other items in
the list. Here, the answer "Yes, severe" was given only 2 points.
People with 8 points or more were regarded as having physical
illness.

Methods

The analyses were performed with the logit regression technique,
which is a log-linear model with a dependent variable *(34)*. With
this type of model, the illness odds in different categories can be
compared with each other simultaneously. The coefficients are
the odds ratio between the odds in each category and the average
odds, represented by the intercept in the model. Thus, the

coefficients can be interpreted as the risk of illness in relation to the mean, i.e. a form of relative risk estimate.

We tried to distinguish between the effects on health of absolute and relative income changes. Two types of confounding factor may affect any relationship between income changes and health, namely, the initial level of income, and the initial health status. To control for these confounders, the logit regression was performed by the inclusion one by one of the indicators of economic change, the position in the income distribution in 1980 and health status in 1980.

Results
Cross-sectional association between income and health
Before looking at the issue of income changes and health, we felt that a study of the pure correlation between income and health status from a cross-sectional perspective might be fruitful. We therefore sorted our sample into ten groups of equal sizes, or interdecile groups, from low to high incomes. Fig. 2 and 3 show the prevalence of physical illness and psychological problems for each interdecile group and for men and women separately. These graphs do not, of course, indicate causality but merely show whether there is a correlation between income and illness in the first place.

To exclude unrepresentative groups, such as healthy young people who were still in education and therefore had low incomes, as well as unhealthy elderly people with relatively low retirement incomes, we restricted our analysis to people aged 35–64. Fig. 2 and 3 show a clear relationship between position in the income distribution and ill health, whether measured as psychological distress or physical illness. This relationship held true both for men and for women but, in the case of physical illness, the relationship seemed to be more pronounced among men. Furthermore, the reverse-J relationship discussed earlier received only weak support in our data. The relationship between illness and income was clearly non-linear, but there was little evidence for an increase in illness among the highest-income groups, except perhaps in the case of psychological distress among men.

This relationship between income and health may be the result of various processes. It may be selective, to the extent that ill people end up with low incomes. If income, in one way or another, causes ill health, this may be the result of the absolute dimension, the relative dimension, or both. In other words, people with low incomes may have worse health because they lack economic resources, or their health may have deteriorated through psychological mechanisms triggered by their income being lower than that of others. To disentangle these possible mechanisms, we turned next to income changes between 1980 and 1990, and health outcome in 1991.

Fig. 2. Percentage of 35–64-year-old men and women reporting psychological distress, by position in the income distribution, in 1991

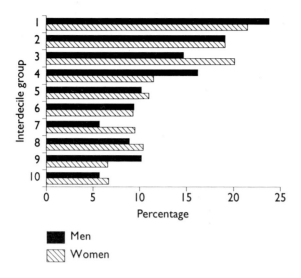

Fig. 3. Percentage of 35–64-year-old men and women reporting physical illness, by position in the income distribution, in 1991

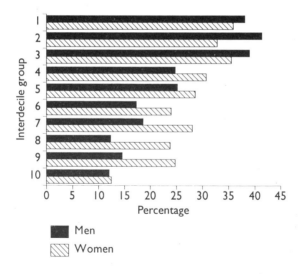

Income change and health

The analyses were done in four steps, producing four models, for men and women separately. In the first model, income change and age were the only independent variables. Thus, the relationship between income change, absolute and relative, could be assessed net of age. In the second model, prior health status was included, to control for income change that was related to health.

In the third model, income change and initial income level were analysed, net of age. The reason for this was that the importance of income change for health was likely to differ according to the initial level of income (measured as interquintile groups). The final model included age, income change, initial income, and initial health status. Since the focus of the analyses was on income and income change, we have not reported the effects on health of age and prior health status in the tables. In all instances, however, these two variables were, as expected, strong predictors of illness.

In Table 7, psychological distress in 1991 is analysed in accordance with these principles (using the labels for income change given in Table 6).

Table 7. Four models showing the odds ratios for psychological distress in 1991 in relation to income change in 1980–1990

Variable	Model 1	Model 2	Model 3	Model 4
Men (N = 957)				
With income change	(0.0396)	(0.1452)	(0.0242)	(0.0384)
A+R+	0.66	0.66	0.53	0.58
A+R0/–	0.99	1.00	1.07	1.07
A0R–	0.90	0.97	0.92	0.97
A–R–	1.70	1.52	1.92	1.68
In interquintile group in 1980			(0.0024)	(0.0611)
1			2.36	1.84
2			1.56	1.40
3			0.98	1.07
4			0.51	0.62
5			0.54	0.59
Women (N = 921)				
With income change	(0.2793)	(0.3620)	(0.1843)	(0.2577)
A+R+	0.79	0.80	0.74	0.75
A+R0/–	0.97	1.01	0.98	1.04
A0R–	1.33	1.30	1.33	1.29
A–R–	0.98	0.95	0.96	1.00
In interquintile group in 1980			(0.0197)	(0.0123)
1			1.15	1.12
2			1.64	1.67
3			0.86	0.90
4			0.54	0.48
5			1.13	1.24

Note: p-values for variable in parentheses.

Starting with men, we found a significant relationship between income change and health (model 1). Among those who experienced an absolute income increase during the 1980s, the ones who lagged behind or remained stable relative to others were less healthy than those who moved upwards in the income distribution. This result supports the hypothesis of a relation between relative income change and health. Among those who had a drop in relative income, on the other hand, those who also experienced an absolute income decrease ran the highest risk of being psychologically distressed. This finding, then, tends to support the hypothesis of a relation between absolute income change and health. These relations remained fairly stable despite the various controls included in the model, although the significance levels changed.

When comparing model 1 with model 3, and model 2 with model 4, the effect of income change on psychological distress became stronger if the initial level of income was controlled for. The interpretation of this somewhat surprising finding is that the relationship between the different types of income change on the one hand and health on the other became blurred, when changes from different income levels were mixed together.

Turning to women, we found a different pattern, but the relationship was insignificant in all four models. Therefore, the reversed order of the A0R– and A–R– categories should not be given that much attention. The odds ratios were quite stable, however, and the differences between models were similar to those found for men. For instance, the relative dimension seemed to be linked with health among those with an absolute income increase, as it was for men. The interquintile variable was also important for women, but the pattern of association was less clear.

Turning next to the impact of income on physical illness, and starting once again with men, Table 8 shows that the pure relation – model 1 – between income change and illness was insignificant. On the other hand, once we controlled for the variable measuring level of income in 1980, which in itself was highly significant, the change variable became significant (model 3). How, then, do we interpret this finding? Obviously, income changes appeared all over the distribution. A rich person, on average, has better health than a poorer person, as shown in Fig. 2. Further, someone with a low income is, statistically speaking, more likely to increase his or her income than someone at the top of the income distribution. Therefore, it is not so surprising that the income change variable did not reach significance in model 1. Thus, when we took the level of income into account (model 3) we got a more accurate picture of the impact of income change.

Again, we find support for the relation between both absolute and relative income change and health. Of the two categories

Table 8. Four models showing the odds ratios for physical illness
in 1991 in relation to income change in 1980–1990

Variable	Model 1	Model 2	Model 3	Model 4
Men (N = 937)				
With income change	(0.4725)	(0.7574)	(0.0379)	(0.1534)
A+R+	0.84	0.88	0.67	0.71
A+R0/–	0.92	0.92	1.06	1.05
A0R–	1.07	1.10	1.00	1.02
A–R–	1.21	1.12	1.40	1.31
In interquintile group in 1980			(0.0000)	(0.0001)
1			1.80	1.81
2			1.43	1.27
3			1.24	1.31
4			0.80	0.87
5			0.39	0.38
Women (N = 912)				
With income change	(0.0862)	(0.1038)	(0.0288)	(0.0565)
A+R+	0.79	0.78	0.71	0.73
A+R0/–	0.93	0.89	0.91	0.87
A0R–	1.37	1.40	1.37	1.41
A–R–	1.00	1.03	1.12	1.12
In interquintile group in 1980			(0.0026)	(0.0506)
1			1.38	1.24
2			1.35	1.17
3			1.16	1.03
4			0.41	0.48
5			1.12	1.40

Note: p-values for variable in parentheses.

with an increasing absolute income (A+R+ and A+R0/–), the ones
who had a relative increase in income as well were in much better
physical health than those who experienced a stable or decreasing relative income. The risk among the latter was almost 60%
higher than among the former, controlling for age and initial
income level. In this case, then, the relative dimension of income
is clearly important. On the other hand, those with both an
absolute and relative drop in income (A–R–) had the highest risk
of physical illness of all men, and their risk was also clearly higher
than among those who only experienced a relative drop (A0R).
This finding supports the importance of absolute income for
health. Consequently, the odds ratios of the income change
variable related to each other in exactly the same way in Table 8
as they did when looking at the effects on psychological distress in
Table 7.

In model 4, which included health status in 1981, the relationship between income change and physical illness turned insignificant again. On the other hand, the odds ratios did not differ much from those in model 3. The odds ratios in models 2 and 3 did not differ much either. The relationship found between income change and health is unlikely therefore to be caused by health selection.

The results for women were to some extent different than those for men. The effect of original income level (interquintile 1980) was, in line with the findings on psychological distress, much less clear. The most plausible explanation for this result is that a married woman's economic situation depends more strongly on the income level of her husband than vice versa. Why the incidence of physical illness was highest among those women who experienced a relative drop but not an absolute drop is harder to explain. We merely note that this finding is once again similar to the one reported on psychological distress (Table 7).

For both men and women, income level in 1980 was highly related to physical illness, although more so for men. Again, the patterns from Table 7 were repeated, both the relative importance of income level in 1980 versus income change, and the sex differences in the health effects of income in 1980. Among men, health status in 1991 improved the higher the income in 1980, while for women the highest interquintile category was unhealthier than the second highest. This clear inverted-J relationship in women became even clearer when health status in 1980 was controlled for. The causes of this sex difference are beyond the scope of this chapter but, since there were fewer women than men in the highest income group (the quintiles being calculated on the basis of men and women combined), the factors behind this health difference may well be found in the sex-segregated labour market and sex differences in wages.

The analyses presented in Tables 7 and 8 show large resemblances. Both the absolute and the relative dimensions seem to be important, although the absolute dimension had a different effect on women than on men. In addition, though, income level 11 years earlier was more important than changes in income, absolute or relative. Whether this should be interpreted as additional support for the importance of absolute income for health, or should rather be taken as evidence supporting relative income as an important factor is another question.

Discussion

These analyses point to income changes, both absolute and relative, as clearly related to physical as well as mental health. Income change was measured between 1980 and 1990, while health was measured in 1991. In addition, health status in 1981 was controlled for, but this did not affect the relationship between income change and health to any substantial degree. In all, then, the findings clearly indicate the importance of income for health status among a sample of working-age individuals, in a country where income differentials are probably among the lowest in the western world *(35)*. Whether this impact is caused by the relative or the absolute dimension of income is less obvious. The results give partial support to both views.

Our findings were much more conclusive for men than for women. The differences between the sexes may be a result of differences in labour market participation, among other things. We would guess, therefore, that an analysis performed on full-time employees only would show more similar patterns for men and women. The use of household income would also possibly produce less divergent patterns between men and women. In further analyses, it might be of interest to include a measure of relative income defined in relation to each person's reference group, rather than in relation to each person's own income history. In an analysis including relative income measured in both ways, Tåhlin *(36)* found larger effects on health from the socially defined measure.

Even when these weaknesses in our study are taken into consideration, we believe that our results help to interpret Wilkinson's findings *(27,28)*. If the absolute dimension of income is important in Sweden, too, then Wilkinson's suggestion, that income distribution and health status are related at a national level through psychological mechanisms, needs further explanation. Maybe it is the absolute income standard among the poorest that is important for public health, rather than general psychological mechanisms triggered by the income distribution *per se*. At any rate, our results, along with those of Wilkinson *(27,28)* and Wennemo *(26)*, among others, suggest that public policies that prevent substantial income loss would be important tools of public health policy. In other words, social insurance schemes that prevent massive income loss in cases of unemployment might be as important as, or even more important than, prevention programmes directed at individuals at risk.

References

1. ENGELS, F. *The condition of the working class in England.* London, Panther Books, 1969.
2. BÄCK, A. *Tal om farsoter som mäst härja bland rikets allmoge* [Discourse on the pestilences that most ravage the kingdom's peasantry]. Stockholm, Vetenskapsakademin, 1765.
3. VÅGERÖ, D. The evolution of health care systems in England, France and Germany in light of 1848 European revolutions. *Acta sociologica,* **26**: 83–88 (1983).

4. FORSDAHL, A. Are poor living conditions in childhood and adolescence an important risk factor for arteriosclerotic heart disease? *British journal of preventive and social medicine*, **31**: 91–95 (1977).

5. FORSDAHL, A. Living conditions in childhood and subsequent development of risk factors for arteriosclerotic heart disease. *Journal of epidemiology and community health*, **32**: 34–37 (1978).

6. BARKER, D.J.P. & OSMOND, C. Infant mortality, childhood nutrition, and ischaemic heart disease in England and Wales. *Lancet*, **i**: 1077–1081 (1985).

7. BARKER, D.J.P. & OSMOND, C. Death rates in England and Wales predicted from past maternal mortality. *British medical journal*, **295**: 83–86 (1987).

8. WAALER, H.T. Height, weight and mortality: the Norwegian experience. *Acta medica scandinavica*, **679**(Suppl.): 1–56 (1984).

9. BARKER, D.J.P. ET AL. Weight in infancy and death from ischaemic heart disease. *Lancet*, **1**: 577–580 (1989).

10. NYSTRÖM PECK, A.M. & VÅGERÖ, D.H. Adult body height, self-perceived health and mortality in the Swedish population. *Journal of epidemiology and community health*, **43**: 380–384 (1989).

11. NOTKOLA, V. ET AL. Socio-economic conditions in childhood and mortality caused by coronary heart disease in adulthood in rural Finland. *Social science & medicine*, **21**: 517–523 (1985).

12. KAPLAN, G.A. & SALONEN, J.S. Socioeconomic conditions in childhood and ischaemic heart disease during middle age. *British medical journal*, **301**: 1121–1123 (1990).

13. LUNDBERG, O. The impact of childhood conditions on illness and mortality in adulthood. *Social science & medicine*, **36**: 1047–1052 (1993).

14. BEN-SHLOMO, Y. & DAVEY SMITH, G. Deprivation in infancy or in adult life: which is more important for mortality risk? *Lancet*, **337**: 530–534 (1991).

15. ELFORD, J. ET AL. Early life experience and adult cardiovascular disease: longitudinal and case-control studies. *International journal of epidemiology*, **20**: 833–844 (1991).

16. ELFORD, J. ET AL. Early life experience and cardiovascular disease – ecological studies. *Journal of epidemiology and community health*, **46**: 1–8 (1992).

17. BARKER, D.J.P. & MARTYN, C.N. The maternal and fetal origins of cardiovascular disease. *Journal of epidemiology and community health*, **46**: 8–11 (1922).

18. BLAXTER, M. *Health and lifestyles*. London, Tavistock, 1990.

19. WHITEHEAD, M. The health divide. *In*: Townsend, P. et al., ed. *Inequalities in health*, 2nd ed. Harmondsworth, Penguin, 1992.

20. TOWNSEND, P. & DAVIDSON, N. Inequalities in health; the Black Report. *In*: Townsend, P. et al., ed. *Inequalities in health*, 2nd ed. Harmondsworth, Penguin, 1992.
21. TOWNSEND, P. *Poverty in the United Kingdom*. Harmondsworth, Penguin, 1979.
22. LUNDBERG, O. Causal explanations for class inequality in health – an empirical analysis. *Social science & medicine*, **32**: 385–393 (1991).
23. SEN, A. The economics of life and death. *Scientific American*, **268**: 40–47 (1993).
24. LE GRAND, J. Inequalities in health: some international comparisons. *European economic review*, **31**: 182–191 (1987).
25. RODGERS, G. B. Income and inequality as determinants of mortality: an international cross-section analysis. *Population studies*, **33**: 343–351 (1979).
26. WENNEMO, I. Infant mortality, public policy and inequality – a comparison of 18 industrialised countries 1950–1985. *Sociology of health and illness*, **15**: 429–446 (1993).
27. WILKINSON, R.G. Income distribution and mortality: a 'natural' experiment. *Sociology of health and illness*, **12**: 391–412 (1990).
28. WILKINSON, R.G. Income distribution and life expectancy. *British medical journal*, **304**: 165–168 (1992).
29. OKUN, A.M. *Equality and efficiency: the big trade off*. Washington DC, Brookings, 1975.
30. KORPI, W. Economic growth and the welfare state: leaky bucket or irrigation system? *European sociological review*, **1**: 97–118 (1985).
31. DUESENBERRY, J. S. *Income, saving and the theory of consumer behaviour*. Cambridge, Harvard University Press, 1949.
32. HIRSCH, F. *Social limits to growth*. Cambridge, Harvard University Press, 1976.
33. ERIKSON, R. & ÅBERG, R., ED. *Welfare in transition. A survey of living conditions in Sweden 1968–81*. Oxford, Clarendon Press, 1987.
34. FREEMAN, D. *Applied categorical data analysis*. New York, Marcel Dekker, 1987.
35. FRITZELL, J. Income inequality trends in the 1980s: a five-country comparison. *Acta sociologica*, **36**: 47–62 (1993).
36. TÅHLIN, M. The value and costs of work: a study of the consequences of wage labour for the individual. *European sociological review*, **5**: 115–131 (1989).

4

Counting the human costs: opportunities for and barriers to promoting health

Margaret Whitehead

Discussions of the effects of economic changes can seem rather abstract because they deal with statistical evidence on whole populations, without reference to how these changes touch individuals in their day-to-day lives. Yet to understand the nature of the link between socioeconomic indicators and health status, we need to know more about what practical opportunities and barriers economic conditions present to people as they strive to promote their own health and that of their families.

This chapter focuses on the way individuals and families live as economic changes unfold, including studies recording what people with inside experience have to say. It starts by taking a long-term view, discussing the positive changes that have occurred in people's health and welfare over the century as a result of economic factors. There have indeed been changes that have made people's lives more comfortable and made it easier for them to keep healthy and avoid disease.

The chapter goes on to consider two economic trends in the last decade that have had a negative effect on people's ability and opportunities to promote their own health: rising unemployment and recession. The result has been poverty for an increasing proportion of the population. The final section considers some implications for research and policy drawn from the studies outlined in the chapter.

Rising living standards: satisfying basic needs

WHO has defined what it calls the prerequisites for health, those conditions that must be satisfied to give people a chance to reach their full health potential, including the following:

people must have the opportunity to satisfy their basic needs in the way of decent food, basic education, safe drinking-water, adequate housing and a useful occupation providing an adequate income *(1)*.

Clearly, in the past 100 years or so, people's opportunities to satisfy some of these basic needs have greatly improved, particularly in industrialized countries. These opportunities are reflected most obviously in increasing life expectancy, brought about by reduced mortality, especially among infants and children under 5 years of age.

This improvement in life expectancy has been attributed to positive economic changes: the increasing wealth and general rise in living standards of populations in countries that have undergone industrial and agricultural development *(2)*. Crucially, countries and local communities had the resources to apply scientific knowledge to improve the conditions under which people lived. According to Doll's analysis *(2)*, the most significant changes in conditions made possible by increasing wealth have reduced the risk of infection and include:

- reduction in the prevalence of malnutrition
- reduction in the prevalence of imperfectly preserved food
- provision of ample water, uncontaminated with faeces
- better housing
- smaller families
- increasing access to education
- increased access to effective preventive and therapeutic health services in the second half of this century.

Summarized in this way, it may sound as though the march of progress towards higher living standards and better living conditions was smooth and uninterrupted. Nothing could be further from reality. Every improvement had to be fought for, policy-makers had to be convinced against the efforts of vested interests and misinformation, and real increases in living standards were slow and intermittent for large sections of the population. In some countries, such as the United Kingdom, industrial growth initially brought with it a serious deterioration in living conditions for a growing proportion of the population. Only when conditions reached crisis point was the impetus sufficient to convince policy-makers that people had to be given access to the prerequisites for health.

Food

As to nutrition, increasing national wealth meant that people had money to buy food and to stave off malnutrition. Over time, food became more plentiful, safer and of better quality, as improved preservation methods and the pasteurization of milk were introduced. Populations were therefore exposed to fewer foodborne pathogens and were in a better nutritional state to resist infection.

It is enlightening to consider just how contaminated and adulterated was the food available to people in the overcrowded towns of nineteenth-century Britain. Even if they could afford to buy food, it might well infect them with disease or parasites, or contain chemicals that would slowly poison them. The practice of padding foods out with cheaper compounds or disguising deterioration was widespread and easy to conceal, as mass production and widespread distribution grew to a massive scale. For example, in 1877, the Local Government Board found that around a quarter of the milk it tested had been watered down or contained chalk (3); 10% of butter, 8% of bread and 50% of gin had copper in them to heighten the colour. Other poisons such as lead, ferric ferrocyanide, strychnine and bisulfate of mercury were all extensively used. A leading reformer on food adulteration found that half the bread he examined had significant quantities of alum added to it (3). This would not poison people directly, but inhibited their digestion and therefore lowered the absorption of nutrients from other foods. The long, but successful, campaigns to introduce pasteurization and safe preservation techniques and to control the adulteration of food went a long way towards giving people the opportunity to obtain a more nourishing, life-enhancing diet.

Drinking-water and housing

In terms of safe drinking-water and adequate housing, many improvements have reduced people's exposure to infection, though things had to get worse before they got better. The rapid urbanization in many countries during the nineteenth century, as people flocked to the towns to find work, caused unprecedented overcrowding, occupational hazards, air pollution and faecal contamination of the water supplies.

In England, the population of many towns doubled in the 30 years from 1801 to 1831, then doubled again in the next 20 years (3). The existing infrastructure could not cope, and it was a daunting struggle for people to avoid disease. Conditions in the cellars of Liverpool illustrate the plight of people in towns at that period. In Liverpool by 1841, some 38 000 people (22% of the population) lived in 8000 subterranean cellars. Each cellar measured about 3 m × 3.6 m and many were more than 1.5 m below ground, but each was home to four or five people. Such dwellings contained no light, heat, ventilation, sanitation or running water – except for the surface water and sewage that flowed down into them from the streets when it rained (3). The wealth of the towns and cities of that period made it possible, after protracted struggles, to provide inhabitants with sewage systems and safer water supplies, and to enact other public health measures to control the vectors of disease and to regulate hazards in the workplace. Outbreaks of cholera, among other epidemics, acted as added spurs to concerted action (4).

Municipal authorities tackled overcrowding in part by slum clearance (including the cellars of Liverpool) and rebuilding programmes, with improved urban design leading to better conditions for the residents. Poor housing policy in some places meant that the intended gains did not always materialize. For example, the rents on renovated properties were sometimes too high for the poor families who used to live in them. In other cases, building standards were too low, creating new problems for the future. Nevertheless, the overall improvements in housing have been impressive, as life-threatening factors in the home environment have been removed (4).

Education and health care

Throughout this century, economic provision has been made to increase access to education and to essential health care and this has also increased people's opportunities to promote their health. For example, the health and welfare of women and children in industrialized countries have benefited greatly from women's greater choice and control over their fertility, brought about by greater access to education and to family planning services (5). The smaller family size and larger intervals between births, resulting largely from effective birth control, have improved the quality of life and survival chances of infants and mothers alike (6). Gauging the scale of this effect is difficult, but one way is to look at the developing countries where women still lack access to knowledge and the means of fertility control. WHO estimates that, if all women who said they wanted to avoid further pregnancies could do so, then at least a quarter of the maternal deaths that occur each year in these countries would be avoided. This would save 150 000 lives per year (7).

Some commentators stress the importance of the direct effect of women's improved economic position, through increasing access to education and paid employment, on many aspects of women's health and welfare (8).

In the latter part of this century, greater access to a wide range of preventive and therapeutic health services has benefited health and welfare. This again has been brought about by policies that remove economic barriers to people using services. For example, in the countries of the Organisation for Economic Co-operation and Development, 6 of the 21 members provided universal cover for hospital costs in 1960, rising to 15 out of 21 by the early 1980s.

All the rest, while not achieving universal cover, had increased public coverage substantially, and the same trend was evident for primary care.

This development has progressively removed the fear of high medical bills and the denial of care when in need, in many industrialized countries. To understand the importance of this development for individuals' peace of mind, it is worth reading the accounts of people who have known that fear. In this extract of an interview originally transcribed in a Scottish dialect, a Scottish woman recalls her childhood in the 1930s.

> At that time, you see, we had to pay for a doctor, when I was little. And that's why I think my mother was so bad because she would not pay for the doctor in case we needed the doctor. With the result her health got worse. If it was in this day an' age now, she would just go to the doctor. But she held off ... because that was a lot of money ... so she sort of suffered in silence you know *(9)*.

Inequalities remain

Most developed countries have also introduced social security schemes during the century, to help people maintain their standard of living during economic crises, following job loss or disability, for example. These schemes have varied in their efficiency and effectiveness, but have prevented the utter destitution and starvation found earlier in the century.

The advances made in satisfying basic health needs in many countries, however, have still not been achieved in poorer parts of the world. In many respects, developing countries face similar conditions to those of industrialized countries 100 years ago. Although more scientific knowledge now exists about the control of both infections and degenerative diseases, these countries do not have the wealth to apply that knowledge. Millions of entirely avoidable deaths continue to occur each year, because of the lack of funds to carry out the public health measures that were possible in wealthy industrialized countries many years ago *(2,4)*.

Of course, over the century, improvements in welfare within countries have not been evenly distributed across the population. Some social groups have benefited faster than others. Some have carried a heavier burden when the economy turned down and have had more limited opportunities as a result. Statistics showing the average for the population as a whole can mask such differences and the continued plight of disadvantaged groups can be overlooked.

Unemployment and states of mind

Many countries are experiencing a rising level of unemployment at present. For some Nordic countries this follows decades of very low rates, while others, such as the United Kingdom, are experiencing a second peak in the space of 10 years.

Between the mid-1970s and mid-1980s, the United Kingdom witnessed a five-fold increase in unemployment so that, by the 1985 peak, 11–13% of the workforce was registered as unemployed and seeking work. This represents over 3 million people. Of these, over 1 million had been unemployed for over a year; 0.5 million for over three years *(10)*. While that rate subsequently declined, a similar peak was reached by early 1993. Given such circumstances, valuable studies have been made of the effects of the changes on health and daily life, though not as many as the magnitude of the issue justifies.

The effects on health of unemployment give cause for grave concern. For a small minority, unemployment appears to lead to an improvement in health. But for the vast majority, it is a devastating experience that can have an effect on physical or, more particularly, mental health *(10)*. Unemployed people often exhibit signs of depression, anxiety, poor self-esteem, neurotic disorders and disturbed sleep and are more likely to commit suicide or attempt to do so. A major study of unemployed people in the United Kingdom found that, 5 months after becoming unemployed, the great majority agreed with the statement that unemployment was "just about the worst thing that ever happened to me" *(11)*.

Unemployment as loss

Over the years, several hypotheses have been put forward as to why unemployment should cause such psychological damage *(12,13)*, summed up neatly by Smith *(14)* as stemming mainly from loss:

- loss of income

- loss of status

- loss of purpose

- loss of social contacts

- loss of a sense of belonging and mattering

- stigma

- humiliation

- reduced scope for making decisions.

That these factors indeed operate in various combinations can be seen from several careful longitudinal studies following individuals' progress after they become unemployed. First, there are studies showing loss of income: the financial consequences of unemployment are often instant and dramatic. Cohort studies of people entering unemployment show that, for many, their income was cut by half as they switched from wages to social security benefits (15,16). The largest British cohort study showed that two thirds of unemployed people had a week's notice or even less, and only 1 in 10 received any form of redundancy payment. Two thirds were aged under 35, and most came from manual or lower service occupations, at the lower end of the pay scale and with low or no educational or technical qualifications (11).

This means that the effects of unemployment were not spread evenly across the population, but fell most heavily on people who already had the lowest income, the least savings, and the worst prospects for future employment. Those who found a job tended to have to take a cut in pay and were at greater risk of being unemployed again within the next two years (11). Unemployment can therefore disrupt people's working lives for years to come.

Shortage of money

Analyses have been made of what it means in practical terms to live on the levels of social security benefits provided for unemployed people. They suggest, for example, that the amount for a couple with two children would be sufficient to provide adequate food and shelter, but not to replace clothes, shoes and furnishings or to participate in social outings or holidays (17). In contrast, other studies have looked at the actual expenditure and consumption patterns of unemployed people. They suggest that they have to cut down on food and public transport, which many people would consider as basic necessities, rather than extras (16,18).

A study of the living standards of different groups of people living on state benefits used a range of indicators, such as whether they ran out of money before the end of the week and whether they ran short of food. Unemployed households were worse off, particularly if they had children, than groups such as pensioners, lone parents and disabled people (19). A third of the children in the households of the 1800 unemployed claimants studied did not have a warm coat and half had only one pair of shoes. Half the couples with children often ran out of money before the end of the week. The same picture emerged from another study that focused on nutrition: unemployed people said that they cut back on food and went without meals when they ran out of cash (20).

Psychological burden

Unemployment reduces social welfare and psychological health. One factor is the increased risk of slipping into poverty, but it is not the only one. The loss of status, the stigma and the humiliation unemployed people have to face add greatly to the burden.

> You feel like a leper, because we live in a work-oriented society. It [unemployment] is not a healthy way to live – you've got to feel you belong in a society.

> Someone dropped a note through my door saying I was a scrounger. It upset me very much. *(18)*.

Unemployed people relate humiliating experiences at the hands of officials dealing with state benefits. The repeated rejection of job applications saps their self-confidence further. A psychiatric study by Fagin & Little followed a group of 22 families through unemployment. They found that some men sank into depression as these negative experiences mounted up, exhibiting sadness, self-blame, feelings of worthlessness and helplessness, sometimes accompanied by impulsive and occasionally violent outbursts *(21)*. Some sought medical advice and they were placed on tranquillizers or mild antidepressants, as were some of their wives.

Change in social behaviour

Unemployment has also been shown to alter people's behaviour, activities and social contacts *(18)*. On balance, they tended to go out less, partly because of lack of money and partly because of the perceived stigma of unemployment. Women in particular mentioned that they missed the socializing that takes place at work, and that they felt cut off from their work friends once they became unemployed. For many, the lack of social activities led to boredom and a greater risk of social isolation.

In the Fagin & Little study, many unemployed men and their wives consumed substantially more cigarettes during the early stages of unemployment. Some men treated smoking as a way of filling the empty hours that stretched out in front of them. For some, it was the main reason for going out of the home if supplies of tobacco were running low *(21)*.

Summing up the findings of several longitudinal studies on the experience of long-term unemployment, White concludes that unemployment tends to corrode social contacts and activities, and leads towards social isolation.

> Exclusion from the world of employment breaks down membership of networks based around employment, while shortage of money leads to a reduction in non-work friendships and wider social and leisure activities *(18)*.

The same studies, however, illustrate the variation in reactions to unemployment. Small groups of people seemed to adapt much better to the experience and did not suffer the same damage. These tended to be older men (for whom there appeared to be less stigma), from higher occupational backgrounds, who had savings and sometimes redundancy payments to cushion the financial effects, space for gardening, and social and cultural hobbies to occupy their time productively.

Sinking into poverty: caring for a family on a low income

Data on changes in income in the United Kingdom over the last decade show how important it is to look at the experience of different groups in the population, instead of just taking the figures for the country as a whole.

Changes in income in the United Kingdom

From 1979 to 1989, real disposable incomes, after paying for housing costs, increased on average by over 30%. Over the same period, however, the poorest tenth of the population experienced a decrease of 6% in their real disposal incomes (22). Even larger differences are seen if the experiences of the richest and poorest households are compared, with increases of 40% for the richest 20% of households (23).

These findings are particularly significant because, throughout the 1980s, economists and politicians argued that there would be a "trickle down effect". This meant that a general growth in the creation of wealth at the top of the social scale would trickle down to benefit everyone, including those at the bottom of the scale. It is now clear that this did not happen in the United Kingdom. When economic changes appeared generally favourable, the rich got richer and there was a general air of prosperity, but the poor were getting poorer.

Furthermore, statistics on disposable incomes indicate only part of the fall in living standards for the poorest sections of the population. Some groups also lost access to certain free goods and services that previously eased their financial situation. For example, some lost entitlement to free or subsidized school meals and to grants for clothing and heating, and gained new responsibilities to pay charges for drinking-water and local taxes. During the 1980s, social security provision changed for other vulnerable groups, including the sick and disabled. A large number of welfare benefits were removed or their real value reduced (24). Large increases in the number of people unemployed, with their families, swelled the ranks of the poor.

The overall result was a doubling of the number of people in the country living in, or on the margins of, poverty over the decade: from 9.4% of the population in 1979 to 21.6% in 1988 (25). This represented 11.8 million people, 3 million of whom were children. Since 1990, the United Kingdom has been experiencing a recession that could make living standards decline for an even greater number of people. The figures to test this prediction, however, take several years to be published and are not yet available.

Effects of changed income on diet

What effect have these economic changes had on the opportunities open to people to promote their health? An examination of personal behaviour and consumption patterns reveals some expected and some paradoxical trends. Throughout the period, low-income groups tended to have a nutritionally poorer diet than more affluent groups. They participated in very little physical activity in their leisure time, yet made less use of free preventive services under the National Health Service. They also continued to have a high prevalence of cigarette smoking (26). The trends in smoking are very striking, as smoking has increasingly become a habit associated with poverty. By 1990, for example, 16% of professional women smoked while 38% of women from unskilled manual households smoked (27). Smoking rates are even higher among women with small children living in deprived areas. Tobacco is the one item of expenditure that low-income households have not cut down on.

To examine the reasons behind these patterns, several different approaches have been taken. Some studies have calculated the resources theoretically required by various households to follow advice on healthy personal lifestyles and assessed whether the actual resources available are adequate. Some have looked at how efficiently available resources are used in different households. Others have explored by qualitative methods the social context in which decisions affecting health are made and the trade-offs that have to be considered.

In the first category, theoretical calculations of what resources people would need to be able to make healthy food choices show that many welfare benefits do not allow people to follow official advice. For example, a recommended diet for a pregnant woman has been calculated to absorb 28% of a couple's income from state benefits (28). An analysis of the special dietary requirements of vulnerable groups such as children, pregnant women, ethnic minorities, and handicapped or elderly people, also concluded that existing benefits for some members of these groups were insufficient for their dietary needs (29). It was shown that the healthy diet recommended by official documents could cost up to 35% more than the typical diet bought by a low-income family (30). In addition, during the 1980s, the price of the foods encouraged in a healthy diet rose more than other, less recommended foods (31).

A major study of household budgets and living standards, undertaken in 1992, calculated the value of a "modest-but-adequate" budget, defined as well above the requirements of survival and well below the levels of luxury. A low-cost budget was also calculated, using cheaper foods and assuming that clothing and other items were made to last much longer. This showed that benefit levels for most types of household were insufficient to reach even the low-cost standard. For example, for a family with two children, the cost of the "modest-but-adequate" budget was over £300 (US $500) per week, the low-cost budget was £141 (US $240) per week, yet the actual amount the family was entitled to from state benefits was £105 (US $180) (32).

Turning to studies of how different households spend their income, low-income households tend to be much more efficient in buying nutrients than their higher-income counterparts, with the exception of vitamin C. As Tim Lang, a food policy analyst, put it recently: "Daily, people at the bottom of the UK social heap perform food miracles" (31). They make meagre resources stretch a long way to feed their families but the problem is that, as calories from fat are cheaper than those from other foods, they tend to buy fattier, less nutritious food products.

Reports made by low-income groups themselves tell a similar story to that of unemployed people discussed earlier. Lack of money is often cited as the reason why low-income families have not bought more fresh fruit and vegetables, even though they say they would like to provide their children with these foods (33). Parents report that they cut down on the food budget and miss meals for themselves, when in financial difficulties. For example, in 1991, a study of 350 families living on low incomes found that one in five parents said they had gone hungry in the last month because they did not have enough money to buy food. Nearly half the parents had gone hungry in the past year to make sure other family members had enough. One in ten children under 5 years of age had gone without food in the previous month and two thirds of children and over half of parents were eating poor diets (34).

Effects of travel costs on health care uptake

Food outlets and health care facilities are increasingly concentrated in central locations. This means that the time and cost of travelling can become important factors in family decisions, particularly in low-income households.

Studies of the uptake of health services, for example, illustrate some of the considerations involved. The National Health Service has expanded some preventive health care services provided free. All sections of the population thus theoretically have a greater opportunity to make use of these services to help promote their health. These include a national cervical cytology service, a national breast-screening programme, and a large expansion since 1990 in health promotion and disease prevention clinics held in general practice surgeries. The rates of uptake of such services, however, continue to show a parallel social gradient with a decrease in uptake with declining socioeconomic group. Hospital outpatient clinics also have quite a high rate of non-attendance, with some health service managers labelling patients as "inconsiderate" and "irresponsible" because they waste health service resources by not turning up *(35)*.

Studies of the practicalities of meeting health care appointments show that many people have to make elaborate arrangements to get to appointments, particularly at distant hospitals. Sometimes the arrangements are so precarious that they break down, or they are so costly in time or money that they threaten to be a serious drain on limited resources. For example, in research in four low-income areas of Liverpool *(35)*, a third of the sample had neither car nor phone. Respondents were asked to describe what was involved for them in meeting a 9.30 a.m. clinic appointment. Their accounts show that they assessed carefully not only what transport was available and how long each leg of the journey would take, but also what arrangements they would have to make for their children or other vulnerable dependents. The trip there and back for a short clinic appointment could often take half a day:

> I had to get 2 buses, and you have to allow for waiting time between buses. It's like nearly half a day's journey just to go to the hospital.

> I had a 2.15 pm appointment and I saw him at exactly 5 to 5. We left here about half past one and got home about quarter past 6. *(35)*.

The respondents often borrowed both care and transport from relatives and friends. In effect, they borrowed time from others, which at some later date they would have to pay back by giving up their own time. They did not call on other people's help lightly, but saved up favours for more urgent occasions for themselves or their vulnerable dependents. Given these factors, it is a wonder that so many actually manage to get to health appointments at all.

The paradox of smoking

The paradox of smoking behaviour in low-income households also needs more detailed investigation. It is a drain on health and meagre household resources, and goes against the careful budgeting and cost saving evidenced in other expenditure and consumption patterns.

Smoking prevalence in the United Kingdom is now highest in unskilled manual households, in unemployed households, and in the poor areas and regions of the country. A particular focus of investigation in recent years has been the lives and circumstances of low-income women, especially those caring for small children at home. This is because the smoking prevalence of women living in such circumstances is extremely high. For example, a community health project in a disadvantaged community in West Belfast, Northern Ireland found that the unemployment rate in the area was 80%, 75% of respondents lived in cold and damp houses, and 89% of women were smokers *(36)*. This association between deprived neighbourhoods and high female smoking prevalence has been confirmed in other parts of the country, especially among mothers of small children *(37,38)*.

What is it about living in such circumstances that encourages such a damaging choice? The conclusion of a recent review of this field *(39)* is that many low-income women use smoking as a coping mechanism – to help them survive in their restricted, depressing environment. Their lives are characterized by skimping and struggling to make ends meet, with all other personal spending stripped to the bone. They have no money to spend on extra food, on clothing or on activities that would take them into the company of other adults and no prospect of a change in the near future. They spend large parts of their days isolated at home with small children, in cramped housing with inadequate play space and no transport. To make this stressful yet monotonous routine bearable and maintain their mental health, some women construct complex ways of coping on their own.

In this context, smoking serves a variety of purposes. For example, it is used as a way of easing tension without leaving their children alone, or as the one "adult" treat they allow themselves, when the rest of their day is concerned with maintaining the wellbeing of other family members. As these low-income mothers explain:

> I always have some [cigarettes] so that in the morning I'm not irritable with the kids *(40)*.

> It's the only thing I do for myself, isn't it? I have to do things for the baby and for my husband, but smoking is about the only thing I can do for myself *(41)*.

These mothers are, in effect, trading off their own physical health in the future against maintaining their mental health and thereby the wellbeing of their family in the present. These are part of the difficult choices and compromises made in the daily struggle to cope with their disadvantaged situations.

Health-related decisions

Of course, low income and poor living environment are not the only barriers preventing people from promoting their health. During the decade, a substantial proportion of the population has experienced an increase in disposable income but has reported difficulties in changing personal lifestyles. The experience and behaviour of prosperous, middle-class families would be a useful area to explore. Surprisingly few such studies exist, but one in Edinburgh interviewed adults and children over a period of 18 months in families selected for their favourable material and social circumstances. The study found that, although they did not have financial stresses, the respondents were faced with another set of difficulties and barriers to following official advice on promoting health. These stemmed from the way modern work patterns and home life are organized, and from their social and childcare obligations *(42)*.

Qualitative studies of how and why people make decisions on health-related issues under differing economic conditions provide much needed insight into the complexities of the processes involved.

Research and policy implications

This chapter concentrates on the evidence from one country, illustrating the kinds of study that have been undertaken to gain a deeper understanding of opportunities for and barriers to promoting health during economic changes. Of course, the results cannot be extrapolated directly to other countries. The unique cultural climate and welfare system in each country make it likely that there will be differences in response to economic changes in different places. But what can perhaps be learnt from these studies is to look at the questions these lines of enquiry have raised and the way these questions can be investigated.

At least three key sets of questions are raised by this work relevant to the current debate. First, there are questions about the distribution of effects across the population. Are the effects spread evenly across social groups, across geographical areas, across age groups, or are some sections of the population affected more than others?

Research on distributional issues in the United Kingdom, for example, reveals that increasing unemployment in the early 1980s fell most heavily on manual workers at the lower end of the pay distribution, who had few if any educational qualifications and were less likely to have savings. Likewise, the fruits of economic growth in the 1980s were unevenly distributed. Although the overall figures indicate a rise in real disposable incomes of over 30% over the decade, these figures mask a deteriorating situation, particularly for families with children in the poorest sections of the population. As a recession set in by mid-1990, these findings emphasize that continued monitoring of the circumstances of different groups will be essential. Studies of how smoking prevalence varied in different communities revealed extremely high rates in areas of multiple deprivation, triggering further lines of investigation.

Second, there are questions about how economic and related policy changes impinge on the practical, day-to-day lives of people as they try to manage their resources and make decisions affecting health, faced by expanding or contracting choices. For example, how do economic changes affect the quantity and quality of food people can buy, their social support networks, their living and working conditions, or their access to health and social services? What factors do they take into consideration when choosing health-damaging or health-enhancing courses of action? How do these factors vary for different groups in the population?

A range of qualitative as well as quantitative approaches has been employed to address such questions. Some studies mentioned above, for example, have calculated how much families of various compositions require to buy the basic necessities for health and wellbeing, and how this compares with what is available to them from state benefits. Others have looked at actual consumption and expenditure patterns. Some have explored the social context in which decisions are made and have drawn on first-hand accounts of people living in various socioeconomic circumstances. Such information can provide a much fuller understanding on which to base health promotion policies, but these studies are few and far between.

Third, such research inevitably raises questions about what can be done about the issues uncovered. Although not touched upon in this chapter, attempts have been made to analyse the policy implications of such studies. For example, the impact of rising unemployment and of poverty on the work of various professionals and agencies has been analysed, revealing gaps in information and in practical skills that urgently need to be filled (43,44). Questions stemming from the communities themselves about what action they can take are starting to come to the fore. Heated debate has been generated about the best policy approach to take on the issue of smoking among women on low incomes, generated by the studies revealing the complexities of living from hand to mouth.

While imaginative interventions are starting to be developed in response to these investigations, they also highlight the many further questions that need to be addressed.

References

1. *Targets for health for all*. Copenhagen, WHO Regional Office for Europe, 1985 (European Health for All Series, No. 1).

2. DOLL, R. Health and the environment in the 1990s. *American journal of public health*, **82**: 933–941 (1992).

3. WOHL, A. *Endangered lives: public health in Victorian Britain.* London, Dent, 1983.

4. ACHESON, D. Health and housing. *Journal of the Royal Society of Health,* **III**: 236–243 (1991).

5. EASTAUGH, V. & WHEATLEY, J. *Family planning and family well-being.* London, Family Policy Studies Centre, 1990.

6. TITMUS, R. *Essays on the welfare state,* 2nd ed. London, Unwin University Books, 1963.

7. ROYSTON, E. & ARMSTRONG, S., ED. *Preventing maternal deaths.* Geneva, World Health Organization, 1989.

8. LEWIS, J. *Women in England 1870–1950.* Brighton, Wheatsheaf Books, 1984.

9. WHITEHEAD, M. *National health success.* London, Association of Community Health Councils for England and Wales, 1988.

10. SMITH, R. *Unemployment and health; a disaster and a challenge.* Oxford, Oxford University Press, 1987.

11. DANIEL, W.W. *The unemployed flow.* London, Policy Studies Institute, 1990.

12. JAHODA, M. *Employment and unemployment.* Cambridge, Cambridge University Press, 1983.

13. WARR, P.B. Twelve questions about unemployment and health. *In*: Roberts, B. et al., ed. *New approaches to economic life.* Manchester, Manchester University Press, 1985.

14. SMITH, R. "Without work all life goes rotten". *British medical journal,* **305**: 972 (1992).

15. MOYLAN, S. ET AL. *For richer, for poorer? DHSS cohort study of unemployed men.* London, H.M. Stationery Office, 1984.

16. WHITE, M. *Long-term unemployment and labour markets.* London, Policy Studies Institute, 1983.

17. BRADSHAW, J. & MORGAN, J. *Budgeting on benefit.* London, Family Policy Studies Centre, 1987.

18. WHITE, M. *Against unemployment.* London, Policy Studies Institute, 1991.

19. BERTHOUD, R. *The reform of supplementary benefit.* London, Policy Studies Institute, 1984.

20. LANG, T. ET AL. *Jam tomorrow?* Manchester, Food Policy Unit, Manchester Polytechnic, 1984.

21. FAGIN, L. & LITTLE, M. *The forsaken families.* Harmondsworth, Penguin, 1984.

22. DEPARTMENT OF SOCIAL SECURITY. *Households below average income: 1979–1988/89.* London, H.M. Stationery Office, 1992.

23. *Hansard,* 16 July 1992.

24. TOWNSEND, P. *The poor are poorer: a statistical report on changes in the living standards of rich and poor in the UK 1979–1989.* Bristol, Statistical Monitoring Unit, Department of Social Planning, University of Bristol, 1991.

25. SOCIAL SECURITY COMMITTEE. *Low income statistics: households below average incomes 1988.* London, H.M. Stationery Office, 1991.

26. WHITEHEAD, M. The health divide. *In*: Townsend. P. et al., ed. *Inequalities in health*, 2nd ed. Harmondsworth, Penguin, 1992.

27. OFFICE OF POPULATION CENSUSES AND SURVEYS. General Household Survey for 1990. London, H.M. Stationery Office, 1992.

28. DURWARD, L. *Poverty in pregnancy*. London, Maternity Alliance, 1984.

29. HAINES, F. & DE LOOY, A. *Can I afford the diet? The effect of low income on people's eating habits with particular reference to groups at risk*. Birmingham, British Dietetic Association, 1986.

30. COLE-HAMILTON, I. & LANG, T. *Tightening belts: a report on the impact of poverty on food*. London, London Food Commission, 1986.

31. LANG, T. Food policy and public health. *Public health*, **106**: 91–125 (1992).

32. JOSEPH ROWNTREE FOUNDATION. *Household budgets and living standards*. York, Family Budget Unit, Joseph Rowntree Foundation, 1992.

33. GRAHAM, H. *Caring for the family*. London, Health Education Council, 1986 (Research Report No. 1).

34. *Poverty and nutrition survey, 1991*. London, National Children's Homes, 1991.

35. PEARSON, M. ET AL. Health on borrowed time? Prioritizing and meeting needs in low-income households. *Health and social care*, **1**: 45–54 (1993).

36. GINNETY, P. ET AL. *A health profile*. Belfast, Moyard Health Group, 1985.

37. HUNT, S. ET AL. *Damp housing, mould growth and health status*. Edinburgh, University of Edinburgh, 1988.

38. GRAHAM, H. Women and smoking in the UK: the implications for health promotion. *Health promotion international*, **3**: 371–382 (1989).

39. *Her share of misfortune: women, smoking, and low income*. London, Action on Smoking and Health, 1993.

40. WELLS, J. & BATTEN, L. Women smoking and coping: an analysis of women's experience of stress. *Health education journal*, **49**: 57–59 (1990).

41. SIMMS, M. & SMITH, C. *Teenage mothers and their partners*. London, H.M. Stationery Office, 1986.

42. BACKETT, K. Health enhancing behaviours in middle-class families. *Health education journal*, **49**: 61–63 (1990).

43. POPAY, J. ET AL. *Unemployment and health: what role for health and social services*. London, Health Education Council, 1986 (Research Report No.3).

44. BLACKBURN, C. *Improving health and welfare practice with families in poverty: a practical guide*. Buckingham, Open University Press, 1992.

5

The effect of social changes on the population's way of life and health: a Hungarian case study

Peter Makara

Hungary has gone through a series of dramatic historical, economic and social changes in the last 50 years. The old post-feudal Hungarian state was buried in the ruins of the Second World War. After the War, the communist take-over of power was followed by the Stalinist storm, the 1956 revolution, the bloody period of reprisals and 30 years of a contradictory lop-sided attempt at consolidation and modernization. The political changes that have taken place since 1988 have brought a sudden and unexpectedly quick transformation to the worlds of politics, economics, society and everyday life.

The effect of the changes over this period is reflected in the morbidity and mortality rates in the population. It might therefore be useful to examine the Hungarian experience more closely. Caution is essential, however, in the theory and method used in the analysis. The changes that have taken place in central and eastern Europe have been so fast and comprehensive that a full scientific picture of society no longer exists. Nor have the full effects appeared yet, so that the analysis must focus on the clearly demonstrable context of the 1980s.

In this chapter, I first outline some features of the transformation process in the region, and then compare the changes in the population's way of life in Hungary with those in Finland, with the help of social indicators. After a review of the main health features, I look at how this links with the effects of the social changes.

The dilemmas of the transition in central and eastern Europe

There was no historical model for the political landslide that struck central and eastern Europe at the end of the 1980s. It was characterized by a complete lack of any theoretical suppositions or normative arguments over who should do what, under what conditions, and with what aims.

One of the most successful branches of research in the social sciences in the last ten years has dealt with the transition to democracy. Three groups of countries have formed the focus of this research:

1. the post-war democracies of Finland, the Federal Republic of Germany,[a] Italy and Japan;

2. the southern European countries that underwent democratization in the 1970s: Greece, Portugal and Spain; and

3. various régimes in South America: Argentina, Brazil, Chile, Paraguay and Uruguay.

The political changes in the former socialist countries differ from these three groups in two fundamental ways. First, central and eastern Europe is dominated by territorial disputes, migration, minority or nationality disputes and occasionally separatist tendencies. Second and more important, the modernization processes in the three groups of countries mentioned were of a political and constitutional kind, while the most urgent task at the end of socialism was the reform of the economy. Whereas in the three groups of countries capital had remained in the hands of its owners, central and eastern Europe faced a very different and more demanding problem: the transfer of the means of production from state ownership to other forms of ownership, and the creation of a new propertied class. Furthermore, politicians have to make and defend these decisions. Unlike in the western democracies, there is no time for a process of learning and gradual maturing in the field of constitutional development and redistributional policy. There is no model to be followed, nor any victorious power that can impose its will from outside.

At the same time, the region has to face the problems of marking out state and population borders, the question of democracy, and the development of an economic system and new ownership structures. This is almost impossible. The market requires the development of democracy, but democracy does not demand the development of the market. Indeed, a sizeable section of the population feels the freedom it has gained is not worth the security it has lost.

A constitutional and democratic political system can only exist if a certain degree of autonomous development has already taken place, and if interest alliances, collective actors and conflict themes have developed. In central and eastern Europe these are often lacking. There are neither the actors, nor the kind of

---

[a] Before the accession of the German Democratic Republic.

problems that can be run through the democratic political machine, but quite the opposite. The lack of a complex civil society means that such themes that do exist, produce conflict but cannot produce compromise. Consequently, as long as the economic basis for a real civil society is lacking, the mass mobilization of the population can only be achieved through nationalist or fundamentalist arguments.

Even if a certain broad social consensus has been reached that the economy should be capitalist – founded on private ownership and determined by goods, services, capital and work – sharp contradictions remain. The basic dilemma is what the "market economy" means in practice, not to mention the "social market". For growth in production can only be achieved if a minority increases its wealth far faster than the majority. The majority may, for an indefinite period, be losers. In the post-socialist countries, the introduction of the market economy is a political plan that can only succeed if it is based on firm democratic legitimacy. In a crisis, however, the population may not consider either democracy or the market economy a particularly desirable prospect (1-7).

Neither economic miracles nor self-sustaining economic growth are to be expected in central and eastern Europe, and any assistance along the lines of the post-war Marshall Plan is unlikely. One possible way to win the time, moral credit and trust that are required for the simultaneous development of democracy and a market economy is to ease the pain of the transformation through continuous and well coordinated internal redistribution. This did not occur even in the former German Democratic Republic, however, amid extraordinarily favourable circumstances.

In the end, the question is whether the key economic groups can be ensured a secure status, and everyone else an unconditional, adequate means of subsistence. No precedent dictates that the welfare state is a precondition for a market economy or for democracy. Clearly, if resources are reserved for social security against the process of "creative destruction", this moderates not only the destruction but also the creation. Thus, there is general pessimism about whether a politically successful privatization of production is possible, alongside a division of goods and services made on the basis of state guarantees. Moreover, social security and protection can easily be branded as ideas inherited from the old régime, which hinders the development of the new economic order and the fruits it is hoped it will bring.

Health in crisis

In central and eastern Europe, the mortality structure has changed significantly since the late 1950s; nowadays, mortality is mainly caused by chronic noncommunicable diseases. A striking feature is the gradual decline in life expectancy at birth (Table 1). No such trend has been observed in any non-socialist country in this period, but similar trends can be observed in all the former socialist countries.

Numerous studies show that this feature derives not from any characteristic of the retired population, but mainly from the enormously high, by international standards, mortality rates among the active population.

Fall in life expectancy

The problem is clearly illustrated by the figures for life expectancy at the age of 30 in the Hungarian population. Some 110–120 years ago, people aged 30 could expect to live on average

Table 1. Life expectancy at birth (in years) in Hungary

Year	Males	Females
1900–1901	36.56	38.15
1920–1921	41.04	43.13
1930–1931	48.70	51.80
1941	54.95	58.24
1949	59.28	63.40
1950	59.88	64.21
1960	65.89	70.10
1965	66.71	71.54
1970	66.31	72.08
1971	66.11	72.04
1972	66.85	72.57
1973	66.65	72.49
1974	66.52	72.38
1975	66.29	72.42
1976	66.60	72.50
1977	66.67	72.99
1978	66.08	72.74
1979	66.12	73.03
1980	65.45	72.70
1981	65.46	72.86
1982	65.63	73.18
1983	65.08	72.99
1984	65.09	73.16
1985	65.30	73.07
1986	65.30	73.21
1987	65.67	73.74
1988	66.16	74.03
1989	65.44	73.79
1990	65.13	73.71
1991	65.02	73.83

Source: Central Statistical Office, Budapest, Hungary.

another 25.4 years. This figure rose over the decades. There was a steady if irregular improvement until 1964, when a peak of 41.7 years of life expectancy was reached for men aged 30. Since that year, mortality rates have worsened. The 1964 figure of 41.7 had fallen below 40 by 1980, and below 38 by the mid-1980s.

Yet, after the War, antibiotics and chemotherapy became widely available in Hungary. Intensive care improved, and all citizens were entitled to health care. The health service far outstripped what had existed in pre-war Hungary. Living standards, including nutrition levels, improved markedly, at least in the 1960s and 1970s. Finally, there was full employment, a factor that should not be underestimated, in terms of its effect on mortality rates. It is, therefore, astonishing to find that mortality rates for adult men in Hungary are lower than in 1941, and almost as low as in the early 1930s.

In certain age groups, the fall in life expectancy is extreme. For example, the mortality rate for 40–44-year-old males rose from 3.4–3.5 per 1000 in the mid-1960s to 7 per 1000 by the early 1990s. In this age group, therefore, mortality is twice is as high today as it was 25 years ago.

Even in western European countries, Canada, Japan and the United States, the mortality rates of the middle-aged groups have been difficult to improve, and for long periods remained stable. This is partly because the rate of 3.4–3.5 per 1000 is very low and hard to push lower. It is also partly because, in these countries, the fall in the mortality rates of middle-aged men stagnated for a period or even rose, although not to the same extent or for as long as in central and eastern Europe.

Thus the middle-aged population's mortality in central and eastern Europe is worsening at an accelerated rate, and includes an increase in so-called avoidable mortality. This is resulting in a declining quality of life and a falling average life expectancy at birth. The active population has to bear the burden of caring for more and more pensioners, a situation exacerbated by the low retirement age. This situation will get worse because of the declining number of births and other related demographic processes. Such are the dangers of this growing burden on the active population that it is called the demographic time-bomb.

The implications of the demographic time-bomb

But the implications of this problem extend beyond demographic, health and sociological issues to economic ones: this phenomenon will affect economic capacity as well.

All these factors have a powerful influence both in Hungary and the other former socialist countries, where social services are broader than in the western democracies. Financing these forms of care is already becoming impossible, and maintaining them would impose such a burden on the economy as to rule out any hope of its becoming internationally competitive. At present, social insurance payments form 60% of wages in Hungary, which is very high by international standards.

At the same time, reducing the level of social support is politically difficult. The burden on the active population is therefore unlikely to change in the immediate future. Yet an increase in life expectancy is an important condition for economic competitiveness.

Numerous studies have dealt with this question recently. They have both presented the shocking facts, and given epidemiological and demographic explanations for the worsening mortality rates. They base their explanation for their observations on individual behaviour and lifestyle factors, having concentrated mainly on risk factors and their connections with mortality. But so far there have been few macrosocial (including economic) approaches to explain this phenomenon.

The approach of these studies has been to emphasize individual responsibility and not take into account social influences on individual lifestyle behaviour. Little attention is given to the circumstances (such as environmental damage or health systems) that can have a serious influence on people's health. But the effects of the political system and the social structure need to be analysed.

It is perhaps unparalleled in history for the mortality rate not to fall for three decades. It would suggest that the decline in average life expectancy in central and eastern Europe cannot be explained at an individual level. An examination of the effects of social changes on the patterns of everyday life is therefore essential.

The rapid changes and crisis in Hungary

Looking at the changes in Hungarian society over the last two decades, one could say that the dramatic last five years represent a separate period, embracing the process of political transition. The precise effect of these years on health cannot yet be documented in the same way as the earlier period has been. The situation that has developed can still be illustrated.

By the end of the 1980s, Hungary's gross domestic product had stagnated; it began to fall, by 4% in 1990 and by 12% in 1991. In 1992, the rate of decline eased to 6%. Unemployment reached 663 000 (13%) by the end of 1992, having risen by 326 000 in 1991 and by 257 000 in 1992. Forecasts for 1993–1994 suggest this figure will rise to 18–20%. There is a growing polarization in incomes, and the population's private savings have shown a marked rise, reflecting domestic uncertainty. The government has used these savings to finance a budget deficit that exceeds 5% of the gross domestic product. Inflation has eased from its peak of

35% in 1991. It fell to 23% in 1992 and 21% in 1993. This is still high and has a basic influence on the conditions for healthy living.

Foreign trade has been a success, as Hungary has managed to adjust to the collapse of its former markets in the eastern bloc. Its convertible currency balance of payments showed a surplus of income in 1992 for the third consecutive year. The balance of payments surplus brought a further fall in the country's net debt.

Changes in consumption

Significant changes have occurred in consumption in Hungary. The Central Statistical Office carries out a biennial survey of 12 000 households. The 1989 and 1991 household budget figures illustrate the main features of the consumption structure in the crisis that has unfolded (Tables 2 and 3).

In 1991, employed households spent on average almost 1.5 times as much on personal expenditure as they did in 1989. Unemployed (mainly pensioner) households spent exactly 1.5 times as much. Since the inflation rate was higher, however, this resulted in a fall in expenditure of 14–17% in real terms.

If one breaks down personal expenditure into current spending and investment, one can see a striking fall in investment between the two years, at current prices. The postponement or cancellation of much investment (which consists of the sums spent on valuable durable consumer goods, building work and property purchases) brought its share of total expenditure down from 22.85% in 1989 to 13.8% in 1991 in employed households, and from 10.5% to 7.5% in pensioner households.

Table 2. Spending per head on the main areas of expenditure

Area of expenditure	Spending per head (Ft)		Percentage change in expenditure
	1989	1991	1989–1991
Foods	21 570	32 620	+ 52.1
Consumer goods	4 626	6 572	+ 42.1
Consumer industrial goods	25 956	37 307	+ 43.7
Clothing	5 676	8 398	+ 48.0
Valuable durables	6 564	5 285	– 19.5
Other	13 715	23 624	+ 72.2
Building work and property purchase	6 983	7 027	+ 0.6
Services	9 261	15 084	+ 62.9
Total personal expenditure	68 396	98 609	+ 44.2

Source: Central Statistical Office, Budapest, Hungary.

Table 3. Percentage breakdown of total personal expenditure

Area expenditure	Percentage of total personal expenditure	
	1989	1991
Foods	31.5	33.1
Consumer goods	6.8	6.7
Consumer industrial goods	37.9	37.8
Clothing	8.3	8.5
Valuable durables	9.6	5.4
Other	20.1	24.0
Building work and property purchase	10.2	7.1
Services	13.5	15.3
Total personal expenditure	100.0	100.0

Source: Central Statistical Office, Budapest, Hungary.

The share of total expenditure that went on food in this two-year period rose from 29.8% to 31.5% in employed households, and fell slightly from 39.8% to 39.5% in pensioner households. This can probably be explained by the fact that pensioner households' disposable income was below average by 1989. Therefore, they had to offset the greater expense of energy, transport, medicines, etc. by reducing the increase in their expenditure on food.

In food consumption, the share of home-produced food tended to grow and of shop-bought food to fall, a trend that began in the early 1980s. The number of items bought shows a smaller fall than the overall cost, meaning that consumption is moving towards cheaper goods.

In general, differences are growing in the expenditure patterns of those on the lowest and highest incomes. In 1991, households on the lowest incomes devoted half their expenditure per head to food and household maintenance, while those on the highest incomes spent less than a third.

Low-income families spend a monthly 2000 Ft (US $20) per head on food, while high-income families spend twice this amount. One should bear in mind that households on a low income tend to have more children, whose needs are smaller than those of adults. Nonetheless, those on low incomes consume annually 35 kg less meat, 16 litres less milk, 50% fewer vegetables and 30% less fruit than those on higher incomes.

Similar differences can be found in the other areas of expenditure, reflecting the differing lifestyles and opportunities that result from income differentials. These can be seen in expenditure on culture, holidays, and household equipment, or in the household's supply of up-to-date durable consumer goods.

A comparison of social changes and lifestyle in Hungary and Finland

Let us turn away from the changes of the last 4–5 years to the decades that preceded them, to a Hungarian-Finnish comparison of changes in lifestyle. The years of close cooperation between statisticians and social scientists in the two countries make this possible (6–10).

Time use surveys

Time use surveys were conducted in Hungary in 1963, 1976–1977 and 1986–1987, and in Finland in 1980 and 1987–1988. The last two in Hungary and the two in Finland were made directly comparable, and detailed comparisons were carried out on their findings (Tables 4, 5 and 6).

Table 4. Time use of men and women between 15–64 years of age

Activities	Hours and minutes (h:min) per day (%)							
	Hungary				Finland			
	1976		1986		1979		1987	
Men								
Employment	6:19	(26)	5:52	(24)	4:25	(18)	4:32	(19)
Domestic work	1:41	(7)	1:44	(7)	1:47	(7)	1:48	(8)
Personal needs	10:28	(44)	10:47	(45)	10:20	(43)	10:08	(42)
Studying	0:18	(1)	0:23	(2)	0:40	(3)	0:33	(2)
Travel	1:16	(5)	1:09	(5)	1:10	(5)	1:21	(6)
Free time	3:58	(17)	4:05	(17)	5:38	(24)	5:38	(23)
Total	24:00	(100)	24:00	(100)	24:00	(100)	24:00	(100)
Women								
Employment	4:13	(17)	3:43	(16)	3:11	(13)	3:18	(14)
Domestic work	4:43	(20)	4:36	(20)	3:43	(16)	3:29	(15)
Personal needs	10:32	(44)	10:47	(45)	10:20	(43)	10:10	(42)
Studying	0:18	(1)	0:20	(1)	0:47	(4)	0:39	(3)
Travel	0:58	(4)	0:55	(4)	1:00	(4)	1:12	(5)
Free time	3:16	(14)	3:39	(15)	4:49	(20)	5:12	(22)
Total	24:00	(100)	24:00	(100)	24:00	(100)	24:00	(100)

Source: Harcsa et al. (9).

Table 5. Time use of employed people

Activities	Hours and minutes (h:min) per day			
	Hungary		Finland	
	1976	1986	1979	1987
Men				
Employment	7:00	6:44	5:51	6:01
Domestic work	1:37	1:41	1:43	1:42
Personal needs	10:17	10:33	10:06	9:55
Studying	0:08	0:04	0:02	0:01
Travel	1:17	1:11	1:07	1:21
Free time	3:41	3:47	5:10	4:58
Total	24:00	24:00	24:00	24:00
Women				
Employment	5:30	5:11	4:48	4:54
Domestic work	4:13	4:05	3:35	3:17
Personal needs	10:15	10:30	10:09	9:56
Studying	0:07	0:04	0:02	0:02
Travel	1:02	0:59	1:00	1:11
Free time	2:53	3:11	4:26	4:38
Total	24:00	24:00	24:00	24:00
Men and women				
Employment	6:17	6:01	5:21	5:29
Domestic work	2:52	2:48	2:37	2:27
Personal needs	10:16	10:32	10:07	9:55
Studying	0:07	0:04	0:02	0:02
Travel	1:10	1:06	1:04	1:16
Free time	3:18	3:29	4:49	4:51
Total	24:00	24:00	24:00	24:00

Source: Harcsa et al. (9).

The major feature of the way of life in Hungary was the very long time spent working. Adding together the amount of time spent in different kinds of work activity (main employment, the secondary economy, building work, housework, travel and education), the total figure for this so-called tied time in the second half of the 1970s was 1½ hours longer in Hungary than in Finland, and in the second half of the 1980s it was an hour longer. This excess was accounted for by the longer time spent in the main employment and the secondary economy or, in the case of women, the longer time spent on housework. The growing participation in the secondary economy is the main reason why the standard of living in Hungary did not fall despite the fall in real wages between 1978 and 1989.

Table 6. Time devoted to paid work by employed people

Activities	Hours and minutes (h:min) per day			
	Hungary		Finland	
	1976	1986	1979	1987
Men				
Primary job	5:57	5:17	4:58	5:12
Income-supplementing non-agricultural work	0:02	0:15	0:04	0:07
Income-supplementing agricultural work[a]	1:01	1:12	0:49	0:41
Total	7:00	6:44	5:51	6:01
Women				
Primary job	4:38	4:32	4:19	4:27
Income-supplementing non-agricultural work	0:02	0:06	0:02	0.06
Income-supplementing agricultural work[a]	0:50	0:34	0:27	0:21
Total	5:30	5:11	4:48	4:54

[a] In Finland, all agricultural work.

Source: Harcsa et al. (9).

The real development of the standard of living in Hungary is very difficult to assess. Up to 1989, real income per head rose. The consumption and stock of consumer durables also rose strongly every year until 1989, although overall consumption began to fall after 1987. Housing stock improved both in quantity and in quality. This would seem to suggest that the standard of living did not drop as much as real wages nor, unlike in Poland, did it crash. The time use surveys would suggest that this was due to the willingness of Hungarian society to work long and hard hours in the secondary economy.

One of the main conclusions of the Finnish-Hungarian time use comparisons of the early 1980s was that Hungarian society had a more work-oriented way of life than did Finnish society. Another important aspect was the highly structured nature of Hungarian society, with its sharp social differences. This was evident chiefly in the large variations in the time devoted to work-like activities, according to sex and social group, as well as between rural and urban communities. Finland by contrast was characterized by less of a variation in these variables.

Official working hours have been cut from 44 to 42 or 40 hours per week in Hungary in the past decade, which has led many analysts to expect an increase in the proportion of free time. But recent research shows that these expectations remain unfulfilled. Only certain groups in the population increased their free time, while most maintained the same time use patterns as before. Studies show that the reduction of time spent in the primary employment has been accompanied by a significant increase in activities that bring in a supplementary income. Consequently, the total amount of work done each year nation-wide has not decreased, although the structure has changed.

The changes in the proportions of time spent on different activities have been greatly influenced by changes in the population structure. For example, the proportion of employed people has decreased significantly in Hungary over the past decade. The same can be said about social groups whose lifestyle rests on a strong tradition of time-consuming everyday work: this is characteristic of the dwindling peasant population in the rural communities. As a result of these two trends, the amount of time the population as a whole, or large segments of it, spends in employment has been greatly reduced.

Small-scale agricultural production, in the form of auxiliary farming, remains the main source of supplementary income in Hungary. Contrary to expectations, this activity is extending to an ever wider stratum of the population. Income-supplementing activities among industrial and white-collar workers have tripled and quadrupled, respectively. Coincidentally, do-it-yourself house construction and related time use have increased to a similar extent.

These tendencies seem to correspond to the trends generally experienced in countries with a market economy: namely the revival of the role of the household economy. Do-it-yourself activities play a major role in this trend. In Hungary, this revival was brought about by motives that differ from those in market economies. In the latter, the process was triggered by changes in values and by the advent of modern household equipment offering a broader range of options. In Hungary, it was more of a subsistence strategy developed in the framework of a shortage economy.

The fact that women with small children spend more time on childcare can also be seen as part of the general trend back to household activities. Women with two children increased the time they spent caring for their children from 64 to 100 minutes per day, and women with three or more children increased their childcare time from 85 to 125 minutes. One can say that this confirms the restoration of the family as an institution. Several functions were being relegated from the home and handed over to outside forces. They are now making their way back into the framework of the family and the home.

In Finland, where the changes have not been as radical, no significant modifications in the internal proportions of time use have occurred. Time use proportions still project the image of a society more oriented towards free time in comparison with Hungary. Nevertheless, the survey shows that Finns use more time in employment during the autumn than they used to. Women do less domestic work than before, while men do more. Students and schoolchildren spend less time on their studies than they did in the late 1970s. People sleep less than before, and meals are more readily taken alongside other activities. The amount of women's free time has increased, while that of men has remained the same. Free time is increasingly dominated by television.

Overall, various trends can be discerned in Finland: the first is towards a differentiation between work and holidays. Work and leisure now fall into two distinct categories; on the one hand, annual leave lasts longer and, on the other, work periods are more intense. The second trend is towards a more equal sharing of domestic work in different population groups. The third trend is towards free time increasingly centred on television.

Reasons for the differences

Modernization has been fundamentally slower in Hungary than in Finland so that, at the time of the economic, social and political transition around 1990, Hungary started off from a lower point. These two countries stood at the same level at the beginning of the century. Economic and social development was faster in Finland in the inter-war period than in Hungary, which found itself falling further behind in the socialist period after the Second World War. The difference in the development of the two countries was especially visible after the 1973 oil crisis. Finland quickly adapted to the new path of economic development under the changed conditions of the world economy. Hungary, on the other hand, did not.

In the field of income and mobility, the Finnish welfare state created roughly the same inequalities (and to the same degree mitigated the former inequalities) as did the socialist régime in Hungary. In Hungarian society, however, a far larger part of an average day is taken up with different kinds of work activity than in Finnish society. In other words, Hungary's socialist road of modernization demanded far greater effort from the population than the Finnish road and with fewer results.

The few figures available on the non-material dimensions of welfare – in a word, on the quality of life – suggest that here the situation is far worse in Hungary than in Finland. Put simply, the Hungarian path of modernization produced far more alienation and a greater breakdown in values and norms than the Finnish road, which was far more balanced. The socialist era can be subdivided into smaller and sharply differing periods, but in terms of quality of life the decline was, it seems, unbroken. Hungary's socialist road of modernization was not only far harder than the Finnish road, but had become totally impassable.

The effect of rapid social and economic changes on people's health

Contemporary science has no comprehensive theory of the inter-relationship between macroeconomic and macrosocial processes and the health of the individual. Numerous factors are well documented, however. Some of these effects relate to the fact of change itself, and to the enforced adjustment to changed circumstances. Others concern the content, character and direction of change. Unfortunately, the last decade in Hungary has seen the plentiful effects of the fall in the standard of living and the worsening of living conditions.

The following factors in social and economic processes can be shown to have had a direct short-term effect on the health of the population:

- changes in the economic environment and living conditions;
- changes and inequalities in the social structure;
- the conflicts and anomie arising from adaptation to the new situation; and
- increased stressful events.

Naturally in the long term, these effects are felt in the context of economic growth, qualitative changes in the natural, social and economic environment, and social transformation.

Changes in food consumption

Of the changes in the economic environment, inflation, the decline in living conditions and the falling standard of living all directly influence the conditions for a healthy life. We have already looked at unfavourable developments in the structure of family budgets; now let us take examples of changes in food consumption (Tables 7 and 8).

The rise in retail food prices in Hungary had a selective effect, hitting worst those who buy an overwhelming proportion of their food: mainly wage and salary earners living in towns and cities, particularly the lower-middle class.

Price rises also had an unequal effect on food consumption patterns. Price elasticity in the consumption of the physiologically more important forms of food generally lies between 0.5 and 1

Table 7. Consumption of selected food items in the home, per head

Food item	1989			1991		
	Bought	Home produced	Total	Bought	Home produced	Total
Meat (kg)	41.4	23.2	64.6	37.4	27.0	64.4
Pork (kg)	11.9	4.9	16.8	10.8	8.5	19.3
Poultry (kg)	9.7	11.5	21.2	8.0	10.2	18.2
Cooked meats (kg)	13.9	5.6	19.5	13.2	6.6	19.8
Eggs (no.)	100	134	234	100	130	230
Milk (litres)	87.8	2.7	90.4	83.2	2.9	86.1
Cheese (kg)	2.0	–	2.0	2.0	–	2.0
Fats (kg)	16.0	5.8	21.8	15.2	6.5	21.8
Lard (kg)	5.7	4.2	9.9	4.7	4.7	9.4
Bread (kg)	71.7	–	71.7	71.8	–	71.8
Potatoes (kg)	23.4	24.8	48.2	24.9	23.5	48.4
Sugar (kg)	24.4	0.3	24.7	20.1	0.5	20.6
Fresh vegetables (kg)	23.5	31.7	55.3	27.5	37.1	64.6
Fresh fruit (kg)	24.1	28.8	52.9	24.4	21.6	46.0

Source: Central Statistical Office, Budapest, Hungary.

Table 8. Changes in consumption of selected food items in the home between 1989 and 1991

Food item	Percentage change in consumption		
	Bought	Home produced	Total
Meat	− 9.7	+ 16.4	− 1
Pork	− 9.2	+ 73.5	+ 14
Poultry	− 17.5	− 11.3	− 15
Cooked meats	− 5.0	+ 17.9	+ 1
Eggs	0	− 3.0	− 2
Milk	− 5.2	+ 7.4	− 5
Cheese	0	–	0
Fats	− 5.0	+12.1	0
Lard	− 17.5	+ 11.9	− 6
Bread	+ 0.1	–	0
Potatoes	+ 6.4	− 5.2	0
Sugar	− 17.6	+ 66.7	− 17
Fresh vegetables	+ 17.0	+17.0	+ 16
Fresh fruit	+ 1.2	− 25.0	− 13

Source: Central Statistical Office, Budapest, Hungary.

(meaning that a 1% increase in price causes a 0.5–1% decrease in consumption). Consumption of the traditional and less healthy foods shows less price elasticity. This means that the effect of price increases on consumption produces, if all else is equal, a greater reduction in healthier, better quality foods than, for example, in white bread or animal fats. If income grows rapidly, the consumption of better quality foods shows an above average increase. Thus, stagnating living standards and rising prices strengthen the traditional nourishment structure and hinder the development of healthier eating patterns.

Naturally, other circumstances also affect food consumption. In the short term, the role of prices in changing the consumption structure is limited.

The Hungarian experience with food prices suggests that price subsidies alone will not encourage healthier eating habits. On the contrary, they represent mainly a form of income redistribution in favour of high-status city and town dwellers.

Changes in behaviour

The last few years have seen a continuous and considerable fall in the population's standard of living, except for the top 10%. At the same time, social conflicts have become more open. Social and health policy has to tackle deprivation, poverty, unemployment, migration and the special plight of ethnic minorities (in Hungary, mainly gypsies). The lower middle classes are in special danger. They have lost the modest but secure means of subsistence they became accustomed to in the 1970s and 1980s, and have slid dangerously down towards poverty.

All statistics indicate the high prevalence of deviant behaviour in Hungary, including high rates of suicide, smoking and alcoholism, and rising crime. As a society's normative regulatedness breaks down, so the problems of social integration increase, and the level of anomie rises.

Society has many different value systems, traditions and coherent adjustment systems (including families and other social networks), offering different means of integrating lives and norms. These value systems, subcultures and social integration processes evolve continuously. As they are linked to prevailing political and intellectual trends, historical turning points become more intense and dramatic.

Often, particular forms of behaviour and attitudes survive the collapse of the political ideas they were linked with. At other times, the entire whole slowly collapses, and the result is anomie. From this, complicated, mixed structures of cohesion emerge. The social strata and subcultures linked to the political ideas that have ended may well survive the crisis through the mediation of other strata and subcultures.

One should bear in mind the kind and number of political and ethical crises that have recently affected the everyday attitudes and value system of central and eastern European societies. It is hardly surprising that the cultures of this region present a peculiar mixture of anomie and integration *(11–15)*.

Amidst the changes up to the end of the 1980s, a more pragmatic adjustment system emerged in the everyday life of eastern European, especially Hungarian, society. This involved a stronger emphasis on consumer values. This brought to the surface an aspect of the anomic disintegration of society: the conflict between generally accepted and culturally supported values and social norms, and the lack of appropriate tools to attain them. There is thus an extreme tension between consumer aspirations and depressed living standards. Society's answer to this was to strengthen its traditional stress management strategy, resulting in greater withdrawal and self-inflicted harm.

The problems of stress management and coping are many. The experience of Hungary shows that a price has to be paid in health and quality of life for the economic crisis and the sudden social changes. This price could, however, be considerably reduced if a comprehensive social policy were worked out. Health promotion in the spirit of the Ottawa Charter, the coordination of social and health policies, the facilitation of community action and the strengthening of social support systems can all help produce better, more effective crisis management. The crisis contains convergent health and economic interests. By building on the interest of individuals and groups through selected priorities, action can be taken to improve levels of health and promote equity.

References

1. ETZIONI, A. Eastern Europe: the wealth of lessons. *Challenge*, **34**: 4–10 (1991).
2. HANKISS, E. *East European alternatives*. Oxford, Clarendon Press, 1990.
3. HABERMAS, J. *Die nachholende Revolution*. Frankfurt am Main, Suhrkamp, 1990.
4. NEE, V. A theory of market transition: from redistribution to markets in state socialism. *American sociological review*, **54**: 663–681 (1989).
5. NEE, V. Social inequalities in reforming state socialism: between redistribution and markets in China. *American sociological review*, **56**: 267–282 (1991).
6. ALESTALO, M. ET AL. *Agricultural population and structural change: a comparison of Finland and Hungary*. Helsinki, Research Group for Comparative Sociology, University of Helsinki, 1987 (Research Report No. 34).

7. ANDORKA, R. ET AL. *Use of time in Hungary and Finland.* Helsinki, Central Statistical Office of Finland, 1983.

8. ANDORKA, R. & HARCSA, I. Economic development and the use of time in Hungary, Poland and Finland. *In*: Harvey, A.S. et al., ed. *Time use studies: dimensions and applications.* Helsinki, Central Statistical Office of Finland, 1986.

9. HARCSA, I. ET AL. *Use of time in Hungary and Finland II: life chances and time use.* Helsinki, Central Statistical Office of Finland, 1988.

10. HARCSA, I. & NIEMI, I. *The use of time in Hungary and Finland, 1986-1987.* Helsinki, Central Statistical Office of Finland, 1989.

11. MERTON, R.K. Social structure and anomie. *American sociological review*, 672–682 (1938).

12. MERTON, R.K. *Social theory and social structure.* New York, The Free Press of Glencoe, 1957.

13. MERTON, R.K. Role sets: problems in sociological theory. *British journal of sociology*, 8: 106 (1957).

14. MERTON, R.K. & NISBET, R.A., ED. *Contemporary social problems. An introduction to the sociology of deviant behavior and social disorganization.* New York, Harcourt, Brace and World, 1961.

15. PARSONS, T. *Action theory and the human condition.* New York, The Free Press of Glencoe, 1978.

6

Social welfare and economic changes

Wolfgang Zapf

The topic of this book can be tackled in a micro-perspective or a macro-perspective, in a short or long time frame. The relationships to be found will sometimes be straightforward and sometimes complex and unexpected. This chapter starts with some empirical analyses that illustrate the variables in question at different levels and in different time frames. Next, I put forward a general argument about the relationship between economic growth and welfare development. This states that mass consumption and the welfare state are both core institutions of modernization and that welfare development is bound up with the success and failure of these institutions. From there, it follows that the future of welfare development in modern societies hinges on the future development of mass consumption and the welfare state. Societies in transition are trying to catch up with mass consumption and the provisions of the welfare state, but intermediate goals may be worth pursuing.

Empirical analyses

The first example is a study of a very elementary relationship between economic changes, social welfare and health at the individual level. The question is how unemployment affects personal health and personal satisfaction. This seemingly straightforward question has stirred serious discussions. The common wisdom is that unemployment is a negative life event that damages personal health. This is borne out in cross-sectional surveys and follow-up studies of special populations, such as workers who lose their jobs through factory closure. Other types of study population, however, may produce different results. For example, Elkeles & Seifert [1] investigated the problem by using the German socioeconomic panel, a representative sample of households, including all their adult members, interviewed every year since 1984. Their study focuses on the first five years (1984–1989) and compares five subpopulations, consisting of people who were:

1. continuously employed;

2. unemployed on the interview day;

3. unemployed for at least six months on the interview day;

4. unemployed for at least twelve months during the whole period; or

5. not seeking work (such as retired people or housewives).

The available health indicators were chronic illnesses, seriously handicapping illnesses, and health satisfaction (Table 1).

Simplifying the many results, the basic message is that unemployed people are less healthy than those in permanent employment. The effect of age on health, however, means people who are not even seeking work are even less healthy. Unemployed people are significantly less satisfied with their health than employed people. There is no proof, however, that unemployment causes bad health. Instead, the explanation may be the healthy worker effect: that less healthy and more handicapped people are overrepresented in groups prone to unemployment. Some observers would see that as an unexpected result, while others take it as proof that the job market works with complex selection criteria. Unemployment has a clear causal effect on the deterioration of health satisfaction, which in itself is a good indicator of individual welfare.

The second example, from my research, is very much on a macro-scale and long-term. It concerns changes in the number of births and marriages in Germany from 1910 to 1992, given separately after 1946 for western and eastern Germany. The starting point for this analysis was the observation that births and marriages fell dramatically in eastern Germany after 1989 and the fall of the Communist régime. Such a dramatic change in basic demographic variables – considered here as indicators of welfare – is undoubtedly an indication of basic changes in the social fabric of society. The long-term comparison of rates might give us some hints of an explanation (Fig. 1).

A first observation is that this 1989–1992 drop really is unique. It is not matched by the decline in births and marriages during the First World War, the Depression or the Second World War, or in western Germany after the baby boom of the 1960s. On the other hand, these earlier swings are so great that a clear effect of social strain and societal stress can be seen on very personal decisions. No one knows, however, all the micro-mechanisms that transform societal stress into individual behaviour. Even in times of heavy fighting, such as in 1942, the number of births rose significantly.

Table 1. Levels of chronic illness, serious health handicap
and health satisfaction, according to respondents' employment status

Employment status	Year	Chronic illness (%)	Serious health handicap (%)	Health satisfaction
				Average score (points 0–10)
Permanently employed	1984	25	7	7.4
	1985	25	6	7.2
	1986	28	6	7.1
	1987	29	6	6.9
	1988	24	–	6.8
Not seeking work	1984	39	17	6.8
	1985	39	17	6.6
	1986	42	18	6.5
	1987	44	17	6.4
	1988	41	–	6.2
Unemployed at interview	1984	27	13	6.7
	1985	27	11	6.8
	1986	33	13	6.7
	1987	41	9	6.5
	1988	31	–	6.3
Unemployed for 6 months at interview	1984	34	15	6.2
	1985	33	16	6.0
	1986	46	15	6.3
	1987	49	13	5.8
	1988	–	–	–
Unemployed for 12 months or more during 1984–1988	1984	35	13	6.7
	1985	32	11	6.7
	1986	34	15	6.8
	1987	37	8	6.6
	1988	32	–	6.4

Source: Elkeles & Seifert (1).

As to the effect of economic changes on birth and marriage, in general the relationship is as expected. The drops in rates are much steeper during war than during recession, however, and the recent decline in births occurred under prosperous economic conditions. The eastern German drop began before the economic downturn and signs of recovery have been observed recently, when the economic crisis has really bitten. The western German baby boom of the 1960s and bust of the 1970s can be explained by changes in social structure: changes in family structure, better education for women and their higher participation in the labour force, and new lifestyles among people without children. The

Fig. 1. Yearly/quarterly percentage change in the number of births, 1910–1992

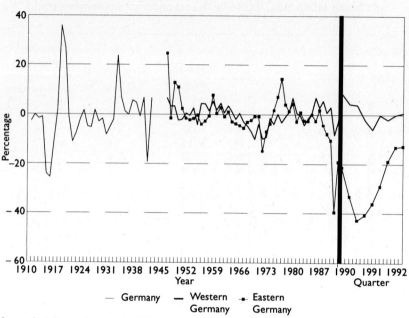

Source: Statistisches Bundesamt (2,3).

1989–1992 drop in births in eastern Germany seems to have a complex aggregate of causes: heavy migration to the west, the rapid overthrow of the eastern German habit of having babies very young in favour of western patterns of later childbirth, combined, however, with a pessimistic outlook and real economic hardships, including rising unemployment and rising living costs.

The third example starts with an analysis of the relationship between economic changes (yearly growth in real gross national product (GNP)) and changes in total expenditure on welfare (yearly growth in real social budget) for western Germany from 1960 to 1990 (Fig. 2). At first sight, the long-term trend shows some similarities: a slight decline in economic growth and a heavier decline in social budget growth but overall significant growth (as most columns are above the zero line) in both GNP and social expenditure. The yearly changes in economic growth and social expenditure seem to have no close correlation, however, even if one allows for a lag-time in social expenditure. Whereas economic growth shows a cyclical pattern with three troughs in three decades, social expenditure shows only one, matching changes in policy: high growth far above economic growth until the mid-1970s, then a slowdown until 1982, with a new expansion during the 1980s. This, indeed, mirrors the story of western German social politics: the big expansion of the early social liberal government after 1969, the slowdown after 1975 and greater leeway during the economic boom of the late 1980s.

Fig. 2. Yearly percentage change in economic and social expenditure growth, at constant prices (1985)

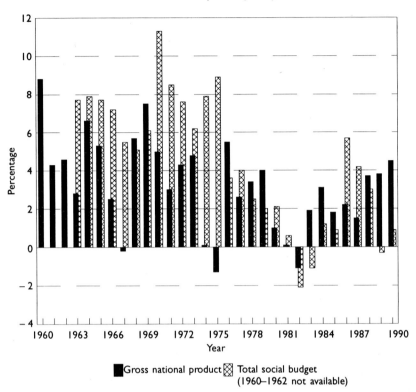

Source: Zahlenbilder (4), Der Bundesminister für Arbeit und Sozialordnung (5).

Other studies and other countries *(6)* confirm that economic changes and social welfare expenditure show no close relationship, especially in the short run and in real terms. The reasons for this are manifold: politicians think in terms of time periods linked to elections as well as to the yearly budget; they look at nominal increases, not constant price calculations; and some of them, not only those in social democratic governments, use social expenditure as stabilizing, anti-cyclical measures. If, however, the relationship between economic changes and social welfare expenditure is rather weak in the short run, it is overwhelming in the long-term development of modern societies. This can be seen in Fig. 2 where the growth between 1960 and 1990 increases GNP in real terms 2.5 fold and social expenditure 3.2 fold. This becomes clearer in the next section.

Economic growth and social welfare

In a long-term perspective, all modern societies show both economic growth and growth in social expenditure. This leads me to a theory of modernization in which the market economy and competitive democracy are innovative institutions, the driving forces of development, and in which mass consumption and the welfare state are integrative institutions. This might be called an institutionalist view. It differs from the view of pure liberals in that it regards the welfare state as a necessary, not just secondary, element of modern societies. It differs from the view of socialists in that it regards mass consumption as the realization of the general upgrading that gives most of the population access to the national output of economy and polity (7). This upgrading can also be measured in terms of general health, most obviously through the increase in life expectancy and the decline of infant mortality.

But my theory is not one of unlimited progress. More subtle health indicators can show the darker side of modern societies. These darker sides become obvious if the wellbeing of the people, integrated by mass consumption and the welfare state, is examined. There is no trend towards an overall increase in happiness in modern societies, and there is a trend towards increasing environmental damage, which harms social welfare. Let us look at just three problems in this sketch of a theory of modern societies, namely, the role of politics during modernization, the economic value of social politics and the expansion of modern welfare states.

In the modernization theory of the 1950s and 1960s, the role of social politics and the establishment of the welfare state were still not fully recognized. T.H. Marshall took the lead with his developmental formula of a sequence of civil rights, political rights and social rights. But he was very sceptical and in 1961 he wrote (8):

> Thus, it seems that the welfare state as we knew it from the 1940s or at least the consensus for it will be strangled by the affluent society. We must perhaps conclude that France and Germany will develop the affluent society without any effort to establish a welfare state.

This was written after western Germany had experienced an enormous expansion in social politics. It reflects the mood of the time, when Galbraith's polemics against public poverty in an affluent society and Rostow's praise of mass consumption were foremost in people's minds (9,10). Rostow came to grips with welfare state development only in the second version of his theory of the stages of economic growth (10), where the stage of a search for new qualities of life follows the stage of mass consumption. Rostow refers to the gradual rise in public expenditure and, even more, in social expenditure, and this is the literature where the contributions to welfare state development started (11). In his model of the political crises of development, Stein Rokkan came close to the welfare state, when he said that political mass participation created the demand for redistribution and the realization of social rights *(12)*. Both Peter Flora *(11)* and Jens Alber *(13)* followed Rokkan's lead. They demonstrated in empirical detail how the general growth of the welfare state became a common feature of European modernization, together with a great variety of national institutional systems. The general growth is explained by the demands that stemmed from industrialization and the dissolution of traditional security systems (the working class problems being only one aspect). The great variations are explained by political differences (despite the common economic growth), such as different degrees of political penetration of the central state and different patterns of party composition and union strength, as well as different speeds and thresholds of economic recovery and growth.

In the discourse about political economy, the role of social politics in economic growth and societal stability was and still is controversial. In Germany, this debate started in the 1920s under the heading of "the economic value of social politics" *(14)*. The idea was to look at social politics not only as an output or cost or end-product, but also as an input or productive force for economic development. Thus, some economists accept the perspective of modernization theory: that social politics has not only compensatory functions ("the ambulance of capitalism"), but preventive and curative functions to stimulate economic development. In recent economics, this debate goes under the label of Okun's conflict, which entails a trade-off between equality and efficiency. An empirical analysis *(15)* gives many examples of cases in which extensive redistribution undermines the productive basis of the economy (such as in Cuba and other Latin American countries), whereas a low level of social protection allows economic growth (such as in authoritarian régimes, but also in Japan and Switzerland). Empirically, however, cases exist in which a low level of social politics accompanies a low level of economic performance. Most interestingly, cases also exist in which developed social politics accompany successful economic performance (such as in western Germany, the Netherlands, Norway and Sweden). Modernization theory considers this last type of case as the most advanced and, in the long run, most successful because it provides personal security, the concertation of leading interests, and consensus for stable industrial relations: "Long-term consistency of a policy makes the difference; policy shocks instead are evil" *(15)*.

Table 2 illustrates the development of the welfare state over time. The general trend of expansion is roughly threefold between 1950 and 1990; significant differences remain between nations, and the gap between leaders and laggards narrows.

To explain this expansion one must distinguish between sociological factors (increasing demands for public protection

Table 2. Percentage of gross domestic product spent on social security
schemes in selected countries, in descending order

Country	1950	1955	1960	1965	1970	1975	1980	1983
Western European								
Sweden	8.3	9.9	11.0	13.6	18.8	26.2	31.9	33.3
Netherlands	7.1	8.4	11.1	15.7	20.0	26.8	28.3	31.9
France	12.6	13.4	13.4	15.8	15.3	24.1	26.7	29.4
Belgium	12.5	13.2	15.3	16.1	18.1	23.6	25.9	28.0
Denmark	8.4	9.8	11.1	12.2	16.6	22.4	29.9	27.9
Italy	8.5	10.0	11.7	14.8	16.3	23.1	21.5	25.7
Western Germany	14.8	14.2	15.0	16.6	17.0	23.5	24.0	24.3
Austria	12.4	12.8	13.8	17.8	18.8	20.2	22.5	24.2
Ireland	8.9	9.3	9.6	10.3	11.6	19.7	20.1	23.5
Norway	5.7	7.5	9.4	10.9	15.5	18.5	20.2	21.9
Finland	6.7	7.6	8.7	10.6	13.1	16.1	18.0	20.6
Great Britain	10.0	9.5	11.0	11.7	13.8	16.2	17.3	20.5
Switzerland	6.0	6.8	7.5	8.5	10.1	15.1	13.7	14.6
Eastern European								
Eastern Germany	–	–	–	12.7	12.3	14.3	15.8	14.7
USSR	–	–	–	11.6	11.9	13.6	14.0	13.8
Other								
United States	–	–	–	7.0	9.5	13.1	12.6	13.8
Australia	–	–	–	8.3	8.0	10.5	10.7	12.4

Source: Alber (16), International Labour Office (17).

after the dissolution of traditional, mostly local security systems),
political factors (growing pressure from working-class parties and
unions on the one hand, and the increasing capacity of state
bureaucracies on the other hand) and, eventually, also the growing self-interest of an enormous welfare bureaucracy. Historically
and empirically, however, it would be equally wrong to say that
all self-help potential has been eroded, as it would to say that the
liberal and conservative parties had no significant role in the
expansion of the welfare state. The consensus seems to be that the
welfare state expansion will not go on forever: that it is a "growth
to limits" (11) because of financial restrictions and built-in
decelerators. The most elementary restriction is the degree of
coverage already attained; others are the features of "economiz-
ing", "juridification" and "bureaucratization" of the big social
service bureaucracies (18).

The future of welfare development in theory

What can be said about the future problems and solutions or
innovations of social politics? Some key concepts of modernization

theory, which assumes endogenous adaptation and innovation forces, may give us some answers.

Growth to limits

Basically, I agree with Flora that the rapid expansion of the welfare state in the 1960s and 1970s is based on unique, transient (i.e. contingent) constellations. Likewise, the present fiscal crisis, like the one in the early 1980s, results from the coincidence of stagflation (inflation, combined with economic stagnation), the demographic wave (of baby boomers entering the labour market), educational expansion (resulting in more people, especially women, wanting to participate in the labour market, in politics and in public life) and the added load of meeting the capital needs of the countries in transition in central and eastern Europe. This constellation is transient. Beyond that, however, are basic trends that Flora (19) has characterized as:

1. the ageing of the population and the necessity of a new contract between the generations;

2. the changing sexual division of labour and the necessity of a new contract between the sexes;

3. the change of values and the necessity of a new contract between the state and the citizens.

If it is correct that no serious political group proposes the dismantling of the welfare state any longer, then political competition will concentrate on the reconstruction of the welfare state at its given high level.

Financing

In the present budget squeeze of modern welfare states and in view of demographic trends, the predictions are that only much higher contributions from all citizens can maintain the present level of services. That would be regarded by many as limiting the welfare state. In the long term, however, significant changes have occurred in the budget of private households as well as of governments. For example, the proportion of private expenditure on food has halved over the last 50 years or so, while food quality has clearly improved. Why not double or even triple the share spent on care of the elderly, over the next 50 years, given modest economic growth? (This would accumulate to a 63% increase if it averaged only 1% per year!) This does not necessarily require the doubling or trebling of contributions to public social security, just innovative combinations of basic social security, private insurance and employee/employer provisions. This would, however, increase both individualization and inequality!

Security and equality

A helpful concept is to regard security and equality as the major
goals of the welfare state: security from the negative consequences
of modernization and equality through the realization of civil,
political and social rights. But these two goals have not been
aspired to at the same rate. Welfare states presumably share more
similar security goals (in terms of coverage, benefits or obligatory
membership) than equality goals. Further, public security policies conform with the parallel development of mass consumption
better than public equality policies would conform with the
broad competition for innovations.

The coming conflicts about the future and the reconstruction
of the welfare state will also centre around the issues of security
and equality. Modernization theory prefers upgrading (or improved status) to redistribution. In other words, a broad increase
in the capacities of individuals and organizations is more important than better mechanisms of distribution. Innovations produce new inequalities, and only their later diffusion achieves new
equilibrium. Various arrangements may attain security but fewer
will attain equality beyond basic equality of opportunity. The
introduction of a basic pension for everyone, which is much
discussed in several countries, would be an instrument more
likely to provide security than equality.

Individualization versus family solidarity

In modernization theory, the pluralization of lifestyles is an
important feature that describes changes in social structure,
beyond class and status groups. Some versions of an individualization theory are much more radical. They postulate the extensive dissolution of intermediate organizations, such as political
parties, trades unions and social clubs, as well as of family and
household bonds. If monadization of this sort really occurs on a
mass scale, it would shake the foundations of the present system
of modern societies. Flora is right in stating (11):

> An equalization of individual rights may even contradict the objec-
> tive of making living conditions and social security for families more
> equal.

The individual–family dilemma was, in fact, recognized in the
early stages of social politics. Modernization theory does not
make normative or functionalist assumptions, such as that severe
anomie is impossible only because it has destructive consequences. On the other hand, modernization theory has no reason
to assume that the present conflict about the redefinition of
women's roles (and men's roles too) should not eventually result
in new institutionalizations, as was the case with earlier class
conflicts. Modern family economics (20) supports this view. The
altruism or solidarity of the nuclear family (of the traditional or

the modern type) can be explained by individual rational choice, if one assumes that the value (utility) of parents depends on the value (utility) of each individual child. This includes the trend to have fewer children per family and to increase the investment in the quality of these fewer children. If the generational bond remains a worthwhile goal and if investments in human capital (in the form of the next generation) are especially profitable, then there are strong economic reasons for the investments to be provided by private households and public programmes. The high proportion of private investment (what sociologists call the placement function of the family) also explains why the family economy continuously reproduces inequalities.

Having, loving, being

The welfare state (or social politics in general) has produced more security and, to a lesser extent, more equality of living conditions. Welfare may mean loving and being *(21)*, in addition to having; in other words, closeness, togetherness, belonging and self-realization. If so, this gives a broader view of welfare that could go beyond all public social politics. I do not want to use such a broad concept of welfare, as this would reduce social politics to minor issues of material supply and care, and limit loving and being completely to a higher level of subjective welfare. On the contrary, loving and being, belonging and self-realization are not merely cognitive, affective states of mind, but have a real material base in social relationships, patterns of access and competence that can be measured and shaped politically. They are an important part of human capital. The earlier writers on social politics wisely pointed to the limits of the bureaucratization, monetarization and juridification of social politics. Instead they base social politics not on one single principle, but on a combination of state responsibility, subsidiarity, solidarity and individual responsibility *(22)*. The future of social politics is to be found in the new definition, operationalization and implementation of these various principles.

The future of welfare development in practice

Welfare development in the sense of mass consumption and the welfare state is unknown outside the modern societies of the western democracy type. Spurts from poverty into industrial society do occur, however, with the population attaining a fair and basic supply of food, housing, education and health. There are several variants of industrial society besides the liberal democratic type: the authoritarian, fascist type and the socialist type. No political dictatorship or command economy, however, has been able in the long run to use the "subjectivity", the creative potential, of the population they themselves have educated. The dominance *(23)* or the evolutionary preponderance of modern societies is based on their capacity to learn, and their legitimation is based on individualization and security, realized through mass consumption and the welfare state. Late capitalism has not collapsed because of a legitimation crisis, but the authoritarian and the socialist systems have.

If this analysis is correct, what is the future of welfare development? Could modern societies based on mass consumption and a welfare state exist all over the world, or at least in many parts of Asia, Africa and Latin America? Could China one day have 600 million cars (the proportion of cars per head of population in western society) or even 250 million (numerically twice as many as in the United States today, although only the proportion per head of eastern Germany)? Or in China could social expenditure alone increase GNP per head thirtyfold? This is unimaginable. It would mean paradise on earth, a worldwide society of luxury and affluence.

How then can one imagine future welfare development and modernization on a worldwide scale? I propose to think in terms of several different socioeconomic civilizations, not in Max Weber's sense as the contrast between Occident and Orient, but in terms of a stratified world society. This society has under-classes and middle classes, below the upper class of the Organisation of Economic Co-operation and Development (OECD) countries, with the chance of upward and downward mobility on a limited scale, as for individuals in a stratified society *(24)*.

For less developed countries, realistic goals of welfare development should be to secure basic levels of nutrition, health, housing and education for their populations. During this process, they must adapt to the demographic transition and build appropriate infrastructures. If developmental politics and foreign aid are to make sense, they should foster self-help and re-invention, not hinder them, and they should avoid the brutal experiences of Manchester capitalism or Soviet collectivization.

The societies in transition in Asia, Latin America and, above all, in central and eastern Europe are confronted with the problem of building the infrastructure for welfare development, i.e. the core institutions of competitive democracy and a market economy. Recent years have shown that there is no evolutionary logic that guarantees automic modernization after the collapse of feudal, colonial or Stalinist structures. Economists talk about the bottlenecks of time and money: the impossibility of catching up with decades of western development in a very few years. Social scientists talk about developmental dilemmas: that, although political freedom has been gained, many of the political, economic and social structures still have to be built before the new freedom can be enjoyed. The societies in transition have the advantage over modern OECD societies that they know what their developmental goals are. They may even enjoy, in some respects, the advantage of backwardness that give them the chance to skip some steps and to learn from others' mistakes. (The modern OECD societies do not have clear developmental goals, but struggle towards an uncertain future, such as the future of the welfare state!) The societies in transition have the disadvantage, however, that modern societies are moving targets *(25)*. If their rates of change, such as economic growth, growth in social expenditure or reduction of infant mortality, are slower than those of the leading modern societies the gap between them will widen.

Conclusion

Overall, one lesson emerges from developmental politics. The tasks of transformation should be divided into the time, space, money and human capital needed. This would reduce these tasks to a manageable size and remove their overwhelming, discouraging magnitude. Uneven development and inequality in space and time should be accepted for a transition period so that a general upgrading can be achieved. Eventually more equality at a higher level will follow, in economic resources, social welfare and health.

References

1. ELKELES, T. & SEIFERT, W. Arbeitslosigkeit und Gesundheit. *Soziale Welt*, **43**: 278–300 (1992).
2. *Bevölkerung und Wirtschaft 1872-1972*. Stuttgart, Statistisches Bundesamt, 1972.
3. *Zur wirtschaftlichen und sozialen Lage in den neuen Bundesländern, April 1993*. Stuttgart, Statistisches Bundesamt, 1993.
4. ZAHLENBILDER. *Konjunkturverlauf in Deutschland*. Hamburg, 1991 (No. 220 000).
5. *Sozialbericht*. Bonn, Der Bundesminister für Arbeit und Sozialordnung, 1990.
6. PFAFF, M. Zur ökonomischen Bedeutung der sozialen Sicherung. *In*: Vobruba, G. *Der wirtschaftliche Wert der Sozialpolitik*. Berlin, Duncker & Humblot, 1989.
7. ZAPF, W. Sozialpolitik in gesellschaftlichen Modernisierungskonzepten. *In*: Vobruba, G. *Der wirtschaftliche Wert der Sozialpolitik*. Berlin, Duncker & Humblot, 1989.
8. MARSHALL, T.H. The welfare state. A sociologial interpretation. *Europäisches Archiv für Soziologie*, **2**: 284–300 (1961).
9. GALBRAITH, J.K. *The affluent society*. Boston, Houghton Mifflin, 1958.

10. ROSTOW, W.W. *Politics and the stages of growth.* Cambridge, Cambridge University Press, 1971.
11. FLORA, P. Quantitative historical sociology. *Current sociology,* **23**: 5–249 (1975).
12. ROKKAN, S. *Citizens, elections, parties.* Oslo, Universitetsforlaget, 1970.
13. ALBER, J. *Vom Armenhaus zum Wohlfahrtsstaat, Analysen zur Entwicklung der Sozialversicherung in Europa.* Frankfurt, Campus, 1982.
14. VOBRUBA, G. *Der wirtschaftliche Wert der Sozialpolitik.* Berlin, Duncker & Humblot, 1989.
15. SCHMIDT, M. Vom wirtschaftlichen Wert der Sozialpolitik. *In:* Vobruba, G. *Der wirtschaftliche Wert der Sozialpolitik.* Berlin, Duncker & Humblot, 1989.
16. ALBER, J. *Wohlfahrtsstaat. In:* Wörterbuch zur Politik. Munich, Piper, 1983, Vol. 2.
17. *The cost of social security.* Geneva, International Labour Office, 1988.
18. ACHINGER, H. *Sozialpolitik als Gesellschaftspolitik.* Hamburg, Rowohlt, 1958.
19. FLORA, P., ED. *Growth to limits.* Berlin, de Gruyter, 1986, Vol. I.
20. BECKER, G.S. Family economics and macro behavior. *American economic review,* **78**: 1–13 (1988).
21. ALLARDT, E. *About dimensions of welfare.* Helsinki, University of Helsinki, 1971 (Research Group for Comparative Sociology, Research Reports No.1).
22. LAMPERT, H. *Sozialpolitik.* Berlin, Springer Verlag, 1980.
23. HONDRICH, K.O. Systemveränderungen sozialistischer Gesellschaften. *In:* Zapf, W., ed. *Die Modernisierung moderner Gesellschaften.* Frankfurt, Campus, 1991.
24. ZAPF, W. Wohlfahrtsentwicklung und Modernisierung. *In:* Glatzer, W., ed. *Einstellungen und Lebensbedingungen in Europa.* Frankfurt, Campus, 1993.
25. ROSE, R. *Making progress and catching up.* Glasgow, University of Strathclyde, 1992. (Studies in Public Policy, 208).

7

The social consequences and connections of economic changes: the case of Finland

Matti Heikkilä
Sakari Hänninen

This chapter has a double perspective. First, it looks at the Finnish economy in crisis from the point of view of government practices and briefly outlines how the depression and welfare state arrangements interact. Then it examines the complicated links between economic change and social welfare. Research on the consequences of economic change, both at the trend level and at the level of annual changes, is discussed in relation to a number of social problems. The research results question many common sense suppositions.

The success story of Finland

It is not long since Finland was congratulated for being the Japan of the Nordic countries. Although basically unfounded, this claim was based on a number of crucial economic indicators: the growth of gross domestic product (GDP), real incomes, domestic demand and investments, and a low level of unemployment. This performance certainly allows Finland to be classified among the nations that have experienced a rapid economic advance.

This conclusion must, however, be tempered by two conditions. First, the cyclical nature of the Finnish economy has made it unstable and vulnerable to inflationary pressures and deficit problems. Furthermore, the capital intensity and the structural one-sidedness of production and exports are linked with relatively low rates of profit and capital productivity. Second, the high growth rates of the Finnish economy, with a real upswing in the 1980s, was largely achieved with foreign loans. In fact, in recent years, Finland has spent much more than it has earned.

The Finnish model

To explain the specific nature of Finland's socioeconomic performance, research has applied the notion of the Finnish model. According to this model, economic regulation in Finland has been characterized by efforts to sustain economic growth – in terms of exports, savings and investments – by directly supporting the price-competitiveness of businesses. Competitiveness is also a primary objective, which has had a strong effect on the management of unemployment and income redistribution, and of social reforms.

The Finnish model is based on the idea that, as a small open economy, Finland's socioeconomic performance depends on its capacity to compete in the world market and that the rest of the economy and society in turn depends on its exporting success.

The government's attempt to sustain the competitiveness of export-oriented businesses despite strong currency fluctuations is best described as devaluation cycles. The political and economic history of post-war Finland is characterized by a series of devaluations of the Finnish currency.

The devaluation of the Finnish mark was a definite, determined policy to compensate for the lack of competitiveness caused not only by inflation but also by inefficiencies in productivity. Devaluations have also been an effective way of redistributing income in favour of the export sector. The fight against inflation has therefore been more or less postponed. Simultaneously, strong interest groups have taken advantage of these devaluations to benefit from the redistribution of income.

The Finnish model is not characterized solely by devaluation cycles. Their disruption of the smooth running of the economy is effectively mitigated by the use of an incomes policy, which has guaranteed consensus through moderate labour market negotiations of a corporatist nature.

The corporatist labour market negotiations have another result. They have enabled the high demand for investments from the capital-intensive sectors of the economy to be met. A policy guarantees that the high rate of savings is channelled to back up large businesses already exhibiting a competitive advantage.

The success of the Finnish economy cannot be explained by the effectiveness of the Finnish model only, in other words, in terms of comparative competitive advantage, a corporatist incomes policy and the concentration of investments. These efforts have also reproduced the traditional weaknesses of Finland's economy, which are a one-sided productive structure and a lack of domestic competition.

To identify further sources of the strength of Finland's post-war socioeconomic performance, we must look at the factors that have stabilized or stimulated the operation of the Finnish model. There are basically three such factors. The first one is the role of Finland's economic exchange with the former USSR, which not only worked as a buffer against market fluctuations but also offered a market for new products. The second factor is linked with the positive contribution of social arrangements, including the social obligations of businesses, to making quality production appear more feasible and attractive than would otherwise have been the case. In other words, the managerial skills of individual producers have been supported by an up-to-date public infrastructure (1). The third factor is the high quality of human capital that has facilitated the translation of existing information into productive innovations. Though Finland has not had a strong supply and circulation of information, the availability of diverse skills among the population has compensated for this. Production has benefited from the enhanced abilities of people who have been both trained at work (learning by doing) and educated at school (learning by learning) (1).

Welfare state arrangements

Finland has been described as a Nordic welfare state, although not unconditionally. Finland achieved a level of expenditure on its welfare state similar to other Nordic countries only in the 1980s. The methods of organizing the welfare state are not necessarily identical, however, in the Nordic countries. The link between societal arrangements and individual welfare is culturally or communally conditioned and historically constituted. The Finnish model is set up to highlight the peculiarities and specificities of Finland as a Nordic welfare state. Many of the social reforms that have consolidated the welfare state arrangements in Finland are vital to the operation of the Finnish model.

The Nordic similarities and Finnish specificities clarify the Finnish welfare state arrangement, which is further influenced by the factors behind Finland's socioeconomic success. Finland's welfare state arrangements can clarify how the effects of economic change, such as rapid growth or a deep recession, are coped with. The effects of economic change first hit the welfare state arrangements, which are a buffer between societal causes and individual effects. By being the first arena in which economic changes are politically translated, specific welfare state arrangements mediate economic effects on the life chances of individuals. In a welfare state such as Finland's, we cannot take it for granted that a directly measurable link exists between economic performance and the social wellbeing of the population.

Particularly in cases of severe economic stagnation, the immediate pressure is directed first against the welfare state arrangements, which have to cope with the negative social effects of fewer opportunities and resources. This fact also explains why expenditure on welfare services is easily picked out as the cause of difficulties, even though the rise in their proportionate share of GDP is only a consequence of external factors.

The signs of crisis

Over the past two decades, Finland has had two severe economic recessions (Fig. 1). Finland's special trading position with the former USSR partly explains how it managed to survive the crisis of the 1970s without severe repercussions. It also partly explains the severity of the present impasse. To understand the specific nature of this crisis, let us carefully trace the sequence of politico-economic events leading up to it.

The present crisis is not just a short-term recession but a deep depression, which has also paralysed the supply-side features of technological innovations and investments. It is not just an economic crisis but also a crisis of management and leadership.

The first signs of recession could be seen in the deterioration of the balance of payments; inflationary pressures were also recognized. These signs were interpreted along traditional lines as signalling the lack of international competitiveness of the Finnish business sector. What was not properly recognized was that the collapse of the Finnish–Soviet economic exchange was imminent and would eventually reposition Finland in the world market.

Though the first crisis signals were interpreted in traditional terms, the measures taken did not follow the usual devaluation cycle. The new monetary policy adopted was strongly deflationary. This policy had been especially designed to meet the demands of the new European currency system. Without much public discussion, Finland liberalized its money markets and affiliated itself with the European exchange rate mechanism by greatly overvaluing the Finnish mark. This opened the doors for speculation.

With prices and expectations still rising, the new monetary policy relied primarily on the markets to take care of the imbalances. The first arguments went something as follows:

> It is quite possible to "finance" a current deficit for a long period under contemporary conditions. Capital can be attracted into a currency (by interest rate changes for instance), since there are now vast sums of financial capital circulating at the world level because of liberalization, so there is less need to be concerned about a current deficit. Thus the "problem" posed by the collapse of [Finland's] exporting potential and subsequent current account

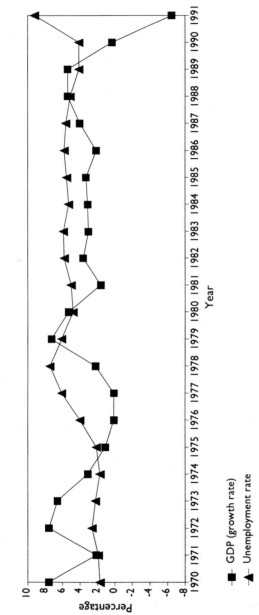

Fig. 1. Annual change in growth of GDP and unemployment rate, 1970–1991

deficit . . . no longer represents a problem because it can be financed fairly easily.[a]

Though disengagement from the devaluation cycle and the fight against inflation were proclaimed as the primary objective even in the 1970s (especially by the Bank of Finland), the policy of a fixed exchange rate for the Finnish mark was not yet really pursued in earnest. The Finnish mark was slightly revalued in 1979, 1980 and 1982, but the devaluations of 1977, 1978 and 1984 had a more profound effect. These measures could not stop the deteriorating trend of the balance of payments that began in 1978.

Despite this development, the Finnish foreign net debt was still only 16% of GDP in 1988. But the Finnish economy was running in a feverish manner, now financed more and more by foreign loans. Shortly after this boom, the Finnish economy ran into severe difficulties and finally into a deep slump in 1991. The result has been a rapid increase in the indebtness of the state, the business sector and private households, which has been met by strict monetary policy, and the weapon of high interest rates.

The new monetary policy advanced by the government and the Bank of Finland could not effectively combat the growing difficulties. Once more, after fierce debate and speculation, the Finnish mark was devalued, although the competitiveness of Finnish businesses had not really deteriorated much. The sudden setback did not, however, mean official abandonment of the tight monetary policy.

Stages of the crisis

The first crucial problem in the present depression is the high foreign indebtness of the Finnish economy – businesses, the public sector and private households – which accumulated in the boom years and was made possible by the liberalization measures. Public sector borrowing to cover the deficit is still escalating rapidly. In 1992, it was 36% of GDP and some calculations suggest it will not reach its zenith until 1998, even with 3% GDP growth and radical annual cuts (in 1994–1995) in public expenditure. In 1992, total output fell by 6.5%. Private investment fell by 19%, which reflects the crisis on the supply side.

Mainly because of the depression, inflation has remained quite low at 4% and the balance of payments has improved slightly. The main result of this development has been a marked increase in the rate of unemployment since 1990. Unemployment has clearly reached a post-war record. In early 1993, 33.3% of the labour force under the age of 25 were unemployed. Unemployment

---

[a] GRAHAME THOMPSON. *Running the economy*. Unpublished paper, 1993.

is the second crucial problem in the present depression and further accentuates the redistribution of possessions in favour of the wealthy that began in the second half of the 1980s.

The causes of the depression are multiple. External factors (such as Finland's position in the world market), internal factors (such as money market supply), and political and government failures have all played a crucial role. This process seems to have advanced in overlapping stages as a chain of difficult events that were signalled first by balance of payments problems, second by indebtness problems, and third by unemployment problems.

Government policy reacted only step by step to this chain of events, thus running into ever more serious difficulties. The credo of the government policy is traditional, but the monetary means have been revised. This policy is based on the assumptions that: first, only growth in the exports and competitiveness of Finnish businesses will regain a market equilibrium and stimulate economic activity, second, only the reduction of public expenditure will cut down the rate of indebtness and, third, only the radical deregulation of labour market relations and incomes policy (including the cancelling of contracts and the reduction of unemployment benefits) will resuscitate the impetus of the supply side. The supply side has actually been strongly supported in Finland since 1977. That year is a landmark in the genealogy of economic policy similar to that of the monetary liberalization right after the middle of the 1980s.

Consequences of the crisis

Although not the real cause of the depression, a crucial effect has been the rise of the relative share of GDP devoted to public expenditure, including social welfare expenditure. The reason is not only the substantial decrease in GDP (in 1991–1992), but also both the massive public support to the private banks struggling with immense losses on bad debts and the high public expenditure to cover the costs of unemployment. This development has radically exacerbated the financial crisis of the welfare state.

The welfare state cannot be labelled – as it often is – as the primary or even central cause of the present crisis. On the contrary, the present crisis and the present government policy seem to question, if not dissolve, many of those social arrangements that have contributed to the stable management of the welfare state through the moral regulation of the economy and the public infrastructure. The present government policy reacts mainly to external compulsions and does not seem able to consider alternative courses of action or to produce social innovations, as happened in post-war Finland. We need not conclude, however, that the existing welfare state arrangements have nothing to do with the origins of the present crisis. The simple fact that the Nordic welfare societies have been both suddenly and severely struck by the present depression demands thoughtful reflection.

To clarify the complex connection between the Finnish welfare state and the present depression, let us look at what happened in the 1980s, when Finland finally adopted the Nordic welfare state model. Careful empirical research shows that, until the end of the 1980s, Finland fared very well, in terms of employment, income equality and lack of poverty. With good reason, these conditions have been linked to the redistributive effect of the welfare state arrangements. This kind of moderately corporatist policy has also, however, cleared the way for strong interest groups – able to harness the mutually reinforcing power of hierarchies, networks and markets – to put forward their specific demands through the established mode of regulation.

The welfare state is economically vulnerable because the well-to-do segments of the population can make accelerating demands without having to take immediate responsibility for the economic setbacks. Further, the extremely high percentage of women engaged in wage labour in the public services sector has, paradoxically, opened the welfare society more to market repercussions. This kind of development, dictated by the demands of the affluent middle classes and supported by their political importance, produced a situation in Finland towards the end of the 1980s in which government measures actually started to redistribute merit-goods and services in favour of the better-off. This development produced an overpriced welfare state whose financial basis started to crumble in the depression of the early 1990s.

At present, the principal socioeconomic consequences of the present depression are clear. They directly impair the material wellbeing of the population in general and of socially weak groups in particular. They are the reduction of incomes, the growing inequality in the distribution of possessions, the high indebtness of private households, and high unemployment. We do not, yet, exactly know what the specific consequences of the public savings are. But we do know that neither the inequality of income distribution, the indebtness of households nor even unemployment are the primary problems that the government policy seeks to cope with. On the contrary, its specific objectives seem to be to challenge inflation, the budget deficit, and public sector debt and to stabilize interest rates and the value of the Finnish mark.

On the complicated links between economic change and social welfare

The connection between economic growth and the social wellbeing of the population in a particular society is a fascinating one. Much depends, naturally, on intermediate aggregate factors that focus on the distributional side of material wellbeing, such as who or which stratum gains the net increase in production. In general, an increase in material wealth along with a proper redistributive policy will lead both to the alleviation of poverty and to a reduction in inequality in income distribution (2,3). The general health status of the population will also improve as all forms of material deprivation in a wide sense are reduced. The question still remains whether the overall growth in GDP also decreases problems related to the quality of life.

Some remarkable empirical work has been carried out in recent years in Finland on this issue and the following trends and results are taken mainly from these sources (4-6).

Kyösti Raunio (4) restricted his data to the period 1950-1977. His idea was to analyse three different although interrelated trends of development simultaneously: (a) the annual growth in GDP, (b) the changes in the level of living, and (c) psychosocial problems. His analysis can be seen as a kind of basis for further work done 10 years later.

Osmo Kontula et al. (5) collected and analysed time series of economic change and social problem indicators over the period 1960-1990. Their approach, however, puts the emphasis more on cross-sectional survey data than on an ambitious study of time-series data.

Lauri Narinen (6) has carefully continued the research path opened by Raunio. Narinen's key questions were the basic ones. How are economic growth and the changes in the unemployment rate related to the number and incidence of certain social problems? Are these links during a period of more stable social and economic development somewhat different from those during a period of rapid transition (as studied by Raunio)?

Economic development in Finland, 1960-1990

Indicators are explanatory variables that tell us something about the general conditions in a particular society. An increase in the level of living on a macro level, such as changes in GDP or the unemployment rate, indicates from different angles the prevailing amount and distribution of material resources in a society. Economic changes can be studied as long-term trends and as short-term fluctuations. Changes in the incidence of different social problems can be handled in the same fashion.

For 40 years, Finland witnessed an unbroken period of economic growth according to the GDP indicator. The year 1991 was the first in post-war history in which GDP actually declined and progress came to a halt. The first period of recession occurred in 1974-1978 and the second (the present one) began in about 1991. Two remarkable peaks appear in the unemployment rate.

The first was in 1977–1979 when the level of 7% was exceeded, and the second is the current one, where the proportion of the total labour force registered as unemployed approaches one fifth.

Indicators of social problems. . .
Different researchers select different indicators to measure the amount and incidence of social problems. In these kinds of study, indicators reflect unmet needs or deviant acts on an individual level, but in the research context they are analysed on the aggregate level. This multi-level construction is important. As Raunio *(4)* has put it:

> . . .welfare problems and deficits appear on an individual level, their causes are at the macro level and the mediating processes act on community level.

Many of the indicators used are the same from one researcher to another. The common denominator of these indicators is that they indicate problems with the quality of life, not with resources in the traditional sense. The time-series data usually cover the following problems: divorce, suicide, alcohol problems (alcohol-related disability pensions and deaths due to alcohol poisoning), mental disorders (disability pensions) and violent crimes (murders).

. . .and economic change
The main indicators of economic change are annual changes in GDP and in the unemployment rate. These two measure different dimensions of the same phenomenon. To allow time for them to have an impact, the effects are measured in three ways – in real time, and logged by one and by two years.

A careful analysis also distinguishes between the overall trend level and the level of annual changes (the fluctuations within the trend). The possible linear dependence between the trend of the problems or effects and the trend of economic change can be studied, as can the connection between short-term (annual) changes (independent of the overall trend).

Growth increases problems
The general result of this research seems to remain unchanged over the periods studied (1950–1977 by Raunio and 1972–1991 by Narinen). Economic growth leads to an increase in most social or psychosocial problems studied on the aggregate level. The only remarkable exception is the development of passive disorders that do not have any significant covariation with the changes in GDP. On the other side, when the focus was moved to the impact on welfare of short-term economic fluctuations, the problems studied tended to decrease during a period of recession.

At first glance, all this seems paradoxical from the point of view of everyday thinking. In Finland, the increased economic prosperity implied that a growing proportion[a] of GDP would be used on social expenditure to prevent social risks. Further, the stressful impact of an economic depression was expected to increase the amount of social problems compared with the average level in a boom period, but that seems not to be the case. Raunio's theoretical explanation stresses the importance of the intermediate level: economic growth particularly promotes the incidence of antisocial behaviour, because it erodes or weakens the ability of the informal society to exert social control and support. This hypothesis could have been true during a very unstable, rapid transition of society from an agricultural stage towards a modern industrial form, as was the case in the 1950s and 1960s. But can this explanation also be valid in the 1970s and 1980s? This can be checked by looking at Narinen's results in a more detailed way *(6)*.

The time-series data from the period 1972–1991 confirm the previous key result. A clear increase in the number of social problems was positively linked with the growth in GDP. The only exception was the mental disorders, as shown by the annual disability pensions granted on the basis of mental problems. This can be interpreted to indicate a kind of passive deviance, where the connection between an individual and the community is weak or cut off. In fact, the only problem indicator that can be explained by the development and variation of the unemployment rate is this very maladjustment: unemployment has a strong negative correlation with mental disorders, even when this impact is measured after one or two years. This means, in simple terms, that during periods of high unemployment the incidence of mental health problems is clearly lower than during low unemployment. The same negative correlation also exists between problem drinking and unemployment. This last finding is reasonable because the level of alcohol consumption per head clearly follows both economic growth and recession.

In the 1972–1991 data, unemployment has a positive regression coefficient only with the number of manslaughters, murders and assaults. A preliminary conclusion (bearing in mind that the discussion so far concerns trend connections) is that there is no connection at the aggregate level between the development of unemployment and social problems (so-called passive mental disorders excluded).

---

[a] In 1970, the GDP share of social expenditure was about 14% and, in 1987, about 26%. The rapid growth in this GDP ratio in 1991 and thereafter was due to the actual decline in GDP.

The influence of short-term economic fluctuations on the annual changes in social problems is in a way more simple. During a boom (when the development of GDP is faster than its average trend and the development of unemployment slower than its average trend), social problems tend to increase, while in a depression they decrease. This connection is exceptionally clear: the GDP indicator shows a positive correlation with every problem indicator, even when the effects are delayed, and the unemployment indicator shows negative correlations with all indicators.

The general picture of the covariation of economic changes and social problems at the population level may seem to be a little controversial, at least where the unemployment factor is concerned. Some reservations and remarks should be made.

The first question concerns the validity of the problem indicators used. One can always argue that indicators such as alcohol-related damage (both to oneself and to others), mental disorders, violence and other forms of illegal behaviour are to some degree signs of the activity of the welfare authorities and the police. This reservation particularly applies to the indicator based on disability pensions. During economic depressions, the general conditions governing the receipt of early pensions, on any grounds, tend to be tightened.

Second, it is hard to believe that high unemployment would not play any decisive role in the rise in severe individual suffering and mental health problems. On the contrary, much evidence suggests that unemployment, and especially its prolongation, increases the risk of other problems. Thus the victims of long-term unemployment are more vulnerable than average (7,8). In the periods studied and reported above, only in 1991 did GDP actually decrease and the unemployment rate reach the current high level. Not enough time-series data are yet available from the period of true economic backlash. This holds especially for the long-term effects of unemployment. Speculations are therefore justified. Let us try to interpret those small signs we have so far of the individual and social consequences of mass unemployment and material deprivation that last for several years.

Unemployment as an individual and societal crisis

During the 1980s, much research was done in Finland on the impact of unemployment on the individual and his or her coping mechanisms. The general impression from this research is that the consequences for the individual were not, generally speaking, as dramatic as one would expect from the public discussions at the time (K. Vähätalo, personal communication, 1993). Signs of passivity or apathy were relatively few; a great majority of the unemployed returned to work without difficulties. This was especially true of young unemployed people (9). Perhaps instead of looking at the general effects of unemployment one should focus on specific life situations and social backgrounds.

The available and relatively rich research data indicate that certain population groups seem to cope more easily than average with unemployment: the young, the elderly, women and, in general, people with a family. On the other hand, single men, the middle-aged and the long-term unemployed seem to have more problems. The relative proportion of the middle-aged unemployed is rising. This group is a kind of risk group in the sense that their experiences of the work ethos, and moral and material obligations overlap most strongly. The economic pressures of employment without compensatory appreciation of its benefits can lead to serious psychological and material problems. About half the unemployed get only the flat-rate benefit (about 2000 Fmk per month) or are even excluded from that owing to the income of the spouse. When this situation becomes chronic, the only option is to apply for means-tested social assistance (supplementary benefit). By 1992, in about 70% of all benefit cases the main reason for dependency was unemployment either with insufficient first-resort benefit or with delayed payments through slow handling by insurance authorities.

One risk group often mentioned among the social concerns are those who drop out of the income-related unemployment security because they have reached the maximum of 500 days of benefit entitlement. For many, this fall is dramatic and will increase the burden of municipal social assistance. Estimates of the number of people facing this drastic financial change varied between 20 000 and 60 000 in 1993. The peak was expected to be reached in the first part of 1994.

On the societal level, the general situation has so far been peaceful or calm, with no large-scale unrest or demonstrations. Nevertheless, some observations can be made about the possible consequences of current economic policies.

According to the government's prevailing economic doctrine, the promotion of exports is the way out of stagnation. This means that the emphasis is on the private sector and that excessive public spending is to be cut heavily. The adoption of this kind of economic pattern will strengthen the areas of production that employ a male labour force. At the same time, the heavy reduction in the public sector and services generally hits the female part of the labour force hardest. In the long run, this can lead to a remarkable loss of sex equality, not only in the working sphere but in society as a whole.

Continuous mass unemployment may also lead to a permanent split in society. One can identify three "sections" of society: the well-off (who are maintaining their positions), the middle class, especially the new middle class (who are in an uncertain and unstable position, and face increased risks) and the traditionally excluded class or "underclass" (which used to be 4-6% of society under stable circumstances). The potential for societal unrest is strongest among those who have never lived without work and/or who lose most in terms of material welfare and social position.

Social peace can be and has been maintained by a relatively high, income-related safety net, combined with training and job creation measures. When (and if) one of these factors disappears, the threat of unrest grows.

References

1. ELAM, M. Markets, morals and powers of innovation. *Economy and society*, **22**: 1-41 (1993).
2. UUSITALO, H. *Muuttuva tulonjako. Hyvinvointivaltion ja yhteiskunnan rakennemuutosten vaikutukset tulonjakoon 1966-1985* [Changing distribution of income]. Helsinki, Tilastokeskus, 1988 (Tutkimuksia 148).
3. GUSTAFSSON, B. & UUSITALO, H. The welfare state and poverty in Finland and Sweden from the mid-1960s to the mid-1980s. *Review of income and wealth*, **36**: 249-266 (1990).
4. RAUNIO, K. *Hyvinvointi ja taloudelliset muutokset* [Social welfare and economic changes]. Turku, Sosiaalipoliittinen Yhdistys, 1983 (Tutkimuksia 41).
5. KONTULA, O. ET AL. Taloudellinen muutos ja terveys [Economic change and health]. Helsinki, VAPK-Kustannus, 1992 (Sosiaali- ja terveyshallituksen, raportti 67).
6. NARINEN, L. *Taloudellinen muutos ja sosiaaliset ongelmat Suomessa 1972-1991* [Economic change and social problems in Finland 1972-1991]. Thesis, Helsinki School of Economics, 1993.
7. RITAKALLIO, V. *Köyhyys ei tule yksin. Tutkimus hyvinvointipuutteiden kasautumisesta toimeentulotukiasiakkailla* [Poverty comes not alone. A study of accumulated welfare deprivation among social assistance recipients]. Helsinki, VAPK-Kustannus, 1991 (Sosiaali- ja terveyshallitus, Tutkimuksia 11/1991).
8. VÄHÄTALO K. *Pitkäaikaistyöttömyyden mosaiikki ja työllisyyslaki* [Long-term unemployment and the law on employment]. Helsinki, Ministry of Labour, 1991 (Työpolittisia tutkimuksia No. 20).
9. SIURALA, L. *Nuorisotyöttömyyden vaikutuksia - myytit ja todellisuus* [On the effects of youth unemployment – the myths and the reality]. Helsinki, Ministry of Labour, 1982 (Työpolittisia tutkimuksia, No. 31).

8

Analysis of the discussion
Laurie McMahon

As explained earlier, the papers on which the chapters of this book are based were presented at a symposium in Helsinki. It was important that the wealth of the material contained in these papers should be used to think about the ways in which national policy-makers might respond to periods of rapid economic change. A workshop design was used so that, after the presentation of each of the papers, participants worked in four small groups to consider the implications for social and health policy. These small groups then reported on their findings in plenary sessions.

To draw all the issues and ideas together into a manageable form, an issues mapping technique developed by the Office for Public Management was used. Each of the points generated in the reports was transferred onto separate pieces of paper. The reports were then broken down into their constituent ideas and issues. These were then clustered and reclustered until dominant themes emerged. The three themes into which the ideas and issues best fitted were:

- values and principles
- information and research
- strategies for action.

Each of these is discussed in more detail below.

Values and principles

The general cluster around the theme of values and principles contained three subclusters: the social meaning of economic change, security and equality as competing principles, and targeting versus universal benefits.

The social meaning of economic change
- National economic performance and the economic activity of individuals, though of great significance, are not synonymous with national and personal identity.

- Strong national culture and the social structures that have evolved from and maintain it are important assets that provide a sense of national wellbeing, especially in times of economic reversal.

- If life is seen as a blend of having, loving and being, then a decline in economic performance probably only has a direct effect on having.

- Rapid economic change has positive aspects, especially the reconsideration of the importance of work roles in social life.

- A shift from the prevailing (economically determined) pattern of social arrangements may be necessary if a new and preferable post-industrial pattern is to emerge.

- The strong negative view of the welfare state as a drain on national resources needs to be countered by a more systemic view. This would suggest that the welfare state serves an important function in holding the fabric of society together in times of rapid economic change, and therefore is a prerequisite to future economic growth.

- Expenditure on health (though not necessarily on conventional health services) should be seen as an economic investment rather than a charge.

- Without the support of the welfare state, it could be more difficult for women to remain in productive employment.

Security and equality as competing principles
- A basic social security system should be maintained for the poor, not just for altruistic reasons, but to maintain social order in times of rapid economic change.

- The effective provision of welfare is essential to smooth out the socially disturbing peaks and troughs of rapid economic change. Such welfare could include income maintenance schemes, subsidies on the price of basic services or the provision of free goods and services.

- A safety net approach, however, could encourage inequality, affect women disproportionately and be used as a lever of direct social control. On the other hand, some inequalities may be inevitable as a precondition of economic growth.

- Equality as a goal of a social welfare system is potentially dysfunctional, especially if the pursuit of equality means that there are compromises on the quality of the safety net (its height above the ground).

Targeting versus universal benefits

- Targeting benefits ensures that the needs of the worst-off are met, though this may have a disproportionately negative effect on women.

- The problem with targeted benefits is that they induce social stigma, which in turn means that they are underused by those they are intended to help.

- Many subpopulations could receive targeted benefits, including young people (to break the generational link in unemployment), recently unemployed young men and the long-term unemployed.

- The argument against targeting is that the poorest (in economic terms) may not be experiencing the most hardship. Taking a relative deprivation approach, the lower-middle classes experience the greatest reversal of fortune. If this argument is accepted, then a strong case is made for maintaining universal earnings-related benefit.

- It is the middle classes that are important in preventing a breakdown in social order.

Information and research

This cluster related to the information and research required to understand the effects of rapid economic change on health, welfare and employment. The general theme broke down into four subclusters: levels of information, types of research, inputs to the policy process and the politics of information.

Levels of information

- Information needs collecting about the health and social effects of economic change at the international, national, community and family levels.

- To improve international information, research bodies need to cooperate more strongly. National differences in the way data are categorized and welfare benefits and services work in different countries must, however, be recognized.

- To improve local and family level information, the community must be involved both in the research design and in the interpretation of results, if researchers are to ascribe proper meaning to their data.

- The way the experience of individuals and communities is assessed needs to be much more creative. More emphasis should perhaps be given to approaches such as social marketing and focus group techniques.

Types of research

- The impact of rapid economic change on the life of the community must be understood. This necessitates a greater use of national household surveys. Surveys of this nature have come under threat in some countries.

- Quantitative analysis of hard, aggregated data needs to be complemented with softer information, if researchers are to understand the dynamics of the changes that lie behind the figures. The case work and social marketing techniques mentioned above can help them do this.

- Softer information also provides a more immediate picture of what is going on. This is increasingly important in times of rapid economic change, since the time needed to develop conventional hard measures may be too long in such circumstances.

- Related to this is the need for a new paradigm for understanding the future, since conventional, hard, extrapolative models become of dubious predictive value in times of rapid social change.

Inputs to the policy process

- If research is to be useful to politicians, then a greater effort needs to be made to improve its user-friendliness and the ease with which it can be assimilated into the policy-making process.

- The research community could give better support to politicians, if the focus of its research were refined by paying greater attention to the comparative cost and benefit of alternative policy options.

- In evaluation of policy options, the narrow expenditure models of costs need to be replaced by a model that includes the true social and economic costs of ill health and unemployment.

- The focus of research needs to shift to include more applied work that monitors and evaluates the impacts and outcomes of policy.

The politics of information

- A determined effort should be made to build strong, positive links between politicians and the research community, if the results of research into the effects of rapid economic change are to be openly and fully debated.

- Any moves to restrict understanding of economic trends and their social impacts, such as the discontinuation of household surveys on civil liberties grounds, must be resisted.

- National research agencies and international agencies such as WHO must forge new alliances, to strengthen their ability to exert greater influence in policy debates.

Strategies for action

Within this cluster, the issues raised did not break naturally into subclusters and so are presented here as an undifferentiated series of points.

- A greater level of private funding of social programmes should probably be accepted. The task of researchers, advisers and policy-makers is to seek the most productive mix of public and private funding, and to try to mitigate the tendency for increases in private funding to increase inequalities.

- Much clearer policy alternatives (for coping with rapid economic change) need to be generated and their links with the political and social values of politicians need to be shown. The values driving social policy need to be much more clearly articulated, including those that underpinned previous welfare systems.

- The effectiveness of social programmes and their relative efficiency need much greater emphasis. Accountability for the performance of programmes needs to be more clearly identified within government and public administration.

- Social programmes must be much more strongly integrated at a strategic and operational level, if the maximum social gain is to be achieved from available resources. One must be able to recognize that changes in one policy area may be caused by changes in another. An example would be recognizing that reducing unemployment benefits may affect the level of expenditure required to cope with the resulting decline in the health of families.

- More particularly, policy-makers should consider the impact on health of investments or disinvestments in other areas of social policy such as transport, education and housing. This more systemic view of health may show that health expenditure is an investment in future economic performance rather than an inhibitor of it.

- To ensure integration happens in practice, policy objectives should probably be made at and for the community level. At this level, integration is much easier to achieve and the motivation for local agencies to work together is highest.

- Action such as service delivery should be based in the community and the community should be involved in the decisions about resource allocation that directly affect it. This enables health and social agencies to build on natural local structures and relationships. It also serves to strengthen community solidarity against individual competitiveness.

- Citizen involvement is a powerful theme. The phrase participative democracy expresses the idea of high levels of devolution to communities. Somewhat paradoxically, for this devolution to occur, it probably has to be deliberately driven by the centre. Allowing local choice of priorities and appropriate programmes would require politicians to trust the people to make the most of national resources.

- Many suggestions for specific initiatives relate directly to Finland. They include:

  - re-examining the mix between cash benefit and retraining benefit for newly unemployed people;

  - treating retraining as a form of employment;

  - developing a secondary labour market that undertakes community and infrastructure development work;

  - reforming the pensions system to make it more flexible, especially in relation to the transferability of pensions;

  - shortening the nationally agreed working week and allowing greater flexibility with the nationally agreed working hours, to draw more people into work;

  - using the mass media to remove the stigma of unemployment; and

  - establishing an early warning system to identify those parts of society where the effects of economic decline have a particularly damaging effect.

Annex

Symposium participants

Seppo Aro	National Research and Development Centre for Welfare and Health, Helsinki, Finland
Jarkko Eskola	Ministry of Social Affairs and Health, Helsinki, Finland
Anni Hakkarainen	Provincial Government of Uusimaa, Helsinki, Finland
Tarja Halonen	Member of Parliament, Helsinki, Finland
Matti Heikkilä	National Research and Development Centre for Welfare and Health, Helsinki, Finland
Sakari Hänninen	National Research and Development Centre for Welfare and Health, Helsinki, Finland
Eniwet Kakuwa	Ministry of Community Development and Social Services, Lusaka, Zambia
Esko Kalimo	Social Insurance Institution, Helsinki, Finland
Mirjam Kalland	Association of Voluntary Health, Social and Welfare Organizations (YTY), Helsinki, Finland
Aulikki Kananoja	National Research and Development Centre for Welfare and Health, Helsinki, Finland
Antti Karisto	Helsinki City Information Management Centre, Urban Studies Department, Helsinki, Finland
Marjaliisa Kauppinen	National Research and Development Centre for Welfare and Health, Helsinki, Finland

Kaj Koskela	Ministry of Social Affairs and Health, Helsinki, Finland
Eero Lahelma	Department of Public Health, University of Helsinki, Helsinki, Finland
Pirkko Lahti	Finnish Association for Mental Health, Helsinki, Finland
Lowell S. Levin	Department of Epidemiology and Public Health, Yale School of Medicine, New Haven, Connecticut, USA
Aki Linden	Pori City Health Department, Pori, Finland
Olle Lundberg	Swedish Institute for Social Research, Stockholm University, Stockholm, Sweden
Kalevi Luoma	Government Institute for Economic Research, Helsinki, Finland
Peter Makara	National Institute for Health Promotion, Budapest, Hungary
Simo Mannila	Rehabilitation Foundation, Helsinki, Finland
Laurie McMahon	Office for Public Management, London, United Kingdom
Veikko Mäkelä	National Research and Development Centre for Welfare and Health, Helsinki, Finland
Risto Pomoell	Health and Social Development Corporation (Hedec), National Research and Development Centre for Welfare and Health, Helsinki, Finland
Ossi Rahkonen	Department of Social Policy, University of Helsinki, Helsinki, Finland
Olavi Riihinen	Department of Social Policy, University of Helsinki, Helsinki, Finland
Arja Rimpelä	University of Oulu, Department of Public Health, Oulu, Finland
Anna Ritsatakis	WHO Regional Office for Europe, Copenhagen, Denmark
Maija Strandström	Association of Finnish Local Authorities, Helsinki, Finland
Ilkka Taipale	Pikkukoskentie 20, Helsinki, Finland

Vappu Taipale	National Research and Development Centre for Welfare and Health, Helsinki, Finland
Jouko Vasama	Association of Voluntary Health, Social and Welfare Organizations (YTY), Helsinki, Finland
Heimo Viinamäki	Kuopio University Hospital, Department of Psychiatry, Kuopio, Finland
Margaret Whitehead	The Old School, Ash Magna, Whitchurch, Shropshire, United Kingdom
Wolfgang Zapf	Social Science Centre, Berlin, Germany
Erio Ziglio	WHO Regional Office for Europe, Copenhagen, Denmark